the healthy gut cookbook

How to Keep in Excellent Digestive Health with 60 Recipes and Nutrition Advice

MARGUERITE PATTEN OBE & JEANNETTE EWIN PH.D.

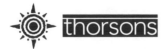

Thorsons

An Imprint of HarperCollins*Publishers*

77–85 Fulham Palace Road,

Hammersmith, London W6 8JB

The website address is: www.thorsonselement.com

thorsons™

and *Thorsons* are trademarks
of HarperCollins*Publishers* Ltd

Published by Thorsons 2004

1 3 5 7 9 10 8 6 4 2

A catalogue record of this book is
available from the British Library

ISBN 0 00 714128 9

Illustration on page 10 by Sarah Wilkinson

Printed and bound in Great Britain by
Scotprint, Haddington, East Lothian

The information contained in this book should by no means be considered as a substitute
for the advice of a qualified medical professional, who should always be consulted before
changing your diet or beginning any new diet, exercise or other health programme.

contents

introduction

According to the Digestive Disorders Foundation, one in ten people suffer pain and distress from illnesses involving the stomach and intestines. These conditions account for approximately one in sixteen deaths in the United Kingdom.

This book is about a remarkable, often misunderstood and frequently embarrassing part of the human body – the gut. The message is simple: eat to take care of your gut and it will take care of you.

While the gut, or digestive system, usually works so well we ignore and often abuse it, things can go terribly wrong. As sufferers of Crohn's disease or irritable bowel syndrome know, a damaged gut can seriously reduce your quality of life. Fortunately, most digestive problems are minor and self-limiting, but even repeated bouts of these can interfere with normal good health and lead to more serious conditions.

Avoiding digestive disasters often requires little more than changing dietary habits. Here is one example of how a poor diet can lead to problems: failure to eat enough high-fibre fruits and vegetables each day can lead to constipation; repeated bouts of constipation may stretch the delicate walls of the lower bowel which, over time, encourages the formation of pockets – or *diverticula*. These pockets may be trouble-free for years. Then infection and inflammation suddenly develop and cause a serious condition known as *diverticulitis*. It might have been avoided. Instead of risking pain and illness, why not follow medical advice and change your diet? When it comes to fruit and vegetables, the 'five-a-day' slogan is a good one.

The Healthy Gut Cookbook aims to change attitudes about diet and the gut. Thanks to Marguerite Patten's story in Chapter 1, concerning her work and her personal experience with irritable bowel syndrome, we have first-hand information about how food has been used over the decades to combat ailments of the digestive system. At the heart of this book are more than 60 recipes Marguerite has written to promote foods that help maintain a healthy gut – and restore one that is flagging.

Written by a nutritionist and health writer, the remainder of the text reflects modern research with contributions from nutritional therapy, traditional Chinese medicine and Ayurveda. (Look for more information about these approaches to healing in the Glossary.) Along with a brief tour of the digestive system and advice on how to maintain a healthy gut, there is a chapter on the special foods that heal and protect the digestive system. A major section describes 20 common and serious illnesses of the digestive system. For each, lists of healing foods and foods to be avoided are provided, along with the names of two or more of Marguerite Patten's healthy-gut recipes.

Information on important related subjects is presented throughout. For example, you will read about how to enjoy eating, which medications affect your gut, tips on food hygiene, and why probiotics is finding wide acclaim. It may come as a surprise that no single diet for a healthy gut is recommended. This is because everyone's needs are unique and change with the ever-shifting circumstances of living. Selecting foods that comfort and balance your digestive system today provides a foundation for a happier and healthier life tomorrow.

If you suffer from a gut disorder and are under a doctor's care, always check with him or her before changing your diet.

So – here's to good eating and a very healthy gut!

Jeannette V. Ewin Ph.D.

one marguerite patten's personal story

When I was young, few people – especially women – used the term 'gut', as it was not considered ladylike. We would have talked about 'stomach' or 'inner' disorders. Nowadays we appreciate the fact that 'gut' is the right word to describe the various internal parts of the digestive system, each of which plays an essential role in keeping us healthy. It is when one or more of these organs is not working properly that we begin to feel unwell.

Throughout most of my life – indeed until quite recently – I have experienced little gut trouble. Over the years, some friends and colleagues have told me of their digestive and internal problems. As I listened to them, I felt extremely relieved that I had not experienced similar complaints. When I think back, the first time I felt really unwell was during pregnancy. I not only suffered from the fairly common morning sickness but I also experienced nausea and some vomiting throughout many days. It was 1942 and I, like so many other people, was worried all the time about the safety of my husband, who was flying in the RAF, and my brother who was at sea. I tried to stay calm and relaxed, as I felt anxiety could only make me feel worse. I had just started work as a food advisor to the Ministry of Food. I held a senior position so had to be efficient and on the ball as I demonstrated ways to make the best use of the relatively limited foods available. I consulted a local doctor, who had never met me before. Although she was sympathetic about my problem, she simply advised me to take sugar in my tea and get as much exercise and fresh air as possible. She gave me an examination and assured me that all was well with the baby.

During the war, doctors were scarce as many younger ones had been drafted into the forces. The doctors left in Britain were very busy, and my problem was a minor one compared to many they had to deal with. The doctor's advice about sweetened tea, which I hated, was actually the catalyst for my interest in the effects of different ingredients upon certain health conditions. My cravings during this time were for highly flavoured ingredients, such as mustard pickles and peppermint sweets, which were difficult to buy on our sparse sweetmeat ration. The flavour I really appreciated was ginger. How I longed for the stem and crystallized ginger of pre-war days. I used ginger, from the ground spice, as often as I could to flavour puddings, cakes and biscuits. Like all expectant mothers, I was allowed a pint of milk daily, and I often flavoured it with ginger to make it more interesting. I was also the recipient of free cod liver oil and concentrated orange juice. It was summertime, so I could follow the doctor's advice and enjoy early evening walks.

After my daughter was born in 1943, the sickness disappeared for a while. However, it returned on a few occasions during 1945, and the condition was diagnosed as a 'grumbling appendix'. This was possibly the reason for the difficulties I had experienced while pregnant. Thankfully, I parted with the appendix later that year and returned to my normal robust health.

By 1945, I was in charge of the Ministry of Food Bureau at Harrods in London. The Food Advisors were qualified home economists who worked throughout Britain. Their role was to help the population make the best use of rations and the limited unrationed ingredients available, and to show people how to prepare enjoyable and nutritious meals. It was not until 1954 that rationing finally ended. The Ministry of Food also employed highly qualified nutritionists and dieticians, and made certain that some of their knowledge was imparted to us. This meant that our demonstrations to the public, and radio talks in my case, incorporated easy-to-follow health information for young and old, as well as suitable recipes.

While at Harrods I extended my interest and knowledge about special diets. At that time the firm employed both a doctor and an experienced nursing sister, both of whom kept watchful eyes on the health of the staff. After my appendix was removed, I had to seek approval to return to work from my own doctor and from the Harrods doctor. If any staff members were on special diets, due to gastric or other medical problems, they had to eat special dishes in a separate part of the staff restaurant, and woe betide them if doctor or sister saw them eating unsuitable meals. I was asked by these two medical experts to provide recipes and suggestions for home cooking for staff members on these special diets. As you can imagine, it was not easy to come up with suitable and inspiring recipes with such limited food resources.

Once I was a recipient of sister's stern instructions. There was a bad epidemic of what was termed 'gastric flu' in and around London and I was one sufferer. I returned to work as soon as possible, still feeling rather delicate. Sister, who had a great interest in cooking and food, came to greet me at the Bureau.

'You look awful,' was her welcoming remark.

'I have felt better,' I replied.

'Go to the grocery department and ask them to sell you a can of Heinz tomato soup. Heat it up and eat it as soon as possible. I know it is scarce but tell them sister says you must have it.'

'I don't like it,' I demurred.

'I am not interested in whether you like it or not – it is what you must have,' was the reply.

I obeyed instructions and must confess the soup did me a lot of good. Sister had worked in America and said she had learned of this simple remedy there. Ever since that time, so long ago, I have recommended the soup to a number of people who were experiencing mild gastric disorders and been told that it did make them feel better. I have never discovered why it is effective, but it may have something to do with the sugars and salt in the soup helping the body regain its normal chemical and fluid balance. You will find more information about 'rehydration' on page 26.

The British Medical Association used to publish a magazine for the general public, and I was engaged as the cookery contributor. Subsequently, I wrote two small booklets for them – one about feeding young children and the second on invalid cookery. In each case I had the benefit of specialist medical advice. Later a publisher commissioned *Marguerite Patten's Invalid Cookery Book*, which was published in 1955.

I began giving television cookery demonstrations for the BBC in 1947 and continued until the early 1960s. In the 1950s I was asked to present, with a doctor, a short series about special diets and dishes for various illnesses. In the last programme of the series, I prepared a tray of dishes suitable for someone who was convalescing. I stressed the importance of presentation to tempt the appetite, as well as the wise choice of food. At that time, all television was live, so there was no opportunity to retake any part of the programme should something go wrong – and something certainly did go awry on that afternoon. Among the dishes on the tray was a rather splendid jelly. I had used extra gelatine to make the jelly set firmly, as studio lighting was very strong and hot in those days. Sadly, while explaining about the dishes and their nutritional importance, there was a 'glug-glug' and my delicious jelly melted and became like a soup, flooding the tray and destroying my elegant meal.

Using extra gelatine is to be avoided in real life. Jellies and other dishes should never be too firm or solid as it takes extra energy to deal with those textures. Someone who is ill, or recovering from an illness, would not be able to cope with such a dish. The recipes in this book have been selected because they look tempting and provide the nutritional needs for various gut ailments. As well as being appetizing, they are easy to eat and digest.

Soon after the outbreak of war, my husband-to-be, Charles Patten, always known as Bob, volunteered for the RAF. He was immediately sent to the Middle East to train as a gunnery officer, after which he took part in operations in that part of the world. One day, the plane in which he was flying crashed. Sadly, there were fatal casualties. Bob was fortunate enough to get out alive and be able to pull injured members of the crew out. He then trekked for 48 hours through the Western Desert and was lucky to meet up with members of the British army. They were able to rescue the rest of the crew. All this happened some time before I met Bob but I learned of the consequences later when he returned to civilian life. In the crash his stomach muscles had been badly strained, and he was not allowed to fly for some time as a result. When we met in Lincolnshire, he was able to return to flying and subsequently carried out many operations.

From time to time, if he was tired or over-strained in any way, he experienced quite severe stomach discomfort, undoubtedly a legacy of the air crash. On some occasion he must have been given slippery elm – or slippery elm tea as it is often called – as he knew of its benefits. I had never heard of it but, when Bob told me about its good effect, I rushed to purchase some and made sure I always had a packet in the house. When Bob had stomach trouble, I used to make up a small helping of slippery elm for him to eat (he preferred it fairly stiff), then we allowed quite a time to elapse before he ate anything else. Slippery elm forms a kind of soothing coating in the stomach, so food eaten afterwards does not give rise to pain. I know, and must stress, that it is not a long-term remedy, as it could hinder the absorption of nutrients. Fortunately, one or two portions of the product did the trick at the time it was needed.

About 12 years ago, we had a more serious matter to deal with. Pills, prescribed by the doctor to alleviate arthritis, gave my husband a perforated stomach ulcer. Obviously he had to have medical treatment for this severe problem. I think our doctor was relieved that I viewed the prospect of providing a special and carefully chosen diet without panic. That state continued throughout the rest of my husband's life.

When people have to watch their diet because of stomach complaints, there are two important points to bear in mind. First, they should not eat in a rush or when tired. In the evening, they should relax and unwind before eating. Second, it may be much wiser for them to eat frequent, lighter meals, rather than a few heavier ones.

I come now to my first-hand experience of gut trouble. It happened in the late autumn of 2001. I was very busy with a number of speaking engagements, articles and books to write. Suddenly, quite out of the blue, I awoke to be faced with the most severe diarrhoea. What on earth could be wrong? I must have dashed to the toilet well over 20 times during the morning and afternoon. Fortunately, someone was available to go to the chemist and get a suitable preparation for me, so I took capsules for the treatment of diarrhoea, following the dosage on the packet. By the evening, these seemed to be making matters slightly better. I was very worried because I would be working away from home over the next few days. I made an appointment to see the doctor on my return and continued 'holding things at bay' with the help of the capsules and a drastic change in my eating habits.

While staying in a hotel I was extremely careful about everything I ate. When I got home, I adapted my diet to omit anything that could make matters worse. I avoided high-fibre ingredients and reduced my previously generous amounts of fruits and vegetables. I was still taking limited doses of the capsules. One day, I remembered a rather simple remedy I had heard of years earlier. It was when I was taking part in a television programme as the cookery expert. On this occasion a doctor was giving a talk on current health matters. While we were chatting together, another of the participants came up to ask her advice. She had bad diarrhoea. Was there anything the doctor could suggest? The studio was a long way from a chemist so she did not have time to buy a suitable remedy.

The doctor's advice was, 'Go down to the canteen and ask them to peel then grate a dessert apple for you. Leave it until it turns brown then eat it. I am sure you will find that a help.'

When the programme had finished, I asked the unfortunate sufferer if the rather unusual apple treatment had proved successful, and she said it had. Remembering this event, I also ate grated apple.

By the time I saw the doctor I was feeling considerably better, although still relying on limited amounts of the capsules. I felt I was more in control of my situation. The doctor looked serious at first and examined me. She was uncertain about what could be the problem, so she arranged for me to see a consultant. In the meantime, she would have tests taken to check whether I had some kind of food poisoning. As I was so busy, I arranged to see the consultant privately to fit in with my work. When I went to the consulting rooms, the gentleman did not give me a great deal of information. He seemed uncertain as to what was wrong. I felt he thought I was making a mountain out of a molehill. By then I had done quite a lot of reading to try and find out more about my condition, so I asked him whether I could have Irritable Bowel Syndrome (IBS).

'Not possible,' was his reply. 'You are far too old for that. Carry on as you are doing and come back in six weeks if you are no better. We will have to consider an exploratory operation.'

I am a member of the Forum on Food and Health at the Royal Society of Medicine. Fortunately, there was to be a day-long meeting on the value of probiotics and their effect on certain ailments. Among the ailments listed in the programme was IBS. I attended the sessions and learned a great deal about probiotics. I also learned that it was quite possible for me to have IBS, even at my advanced age, which was 86 at the time. On my return visit to my doctor I explained about this theory. The tests had shown I had no sign of food poisoning. The doctor by then had considered that it could be a case of IBS. Because I am basically very healthy, I think I have had it fairly mildly, with none of the pain that many people experience. The doctor stated that I had followed the right regime up to that point, and gave me a prescription for suitable capsules in case they were needed in the future. I never take these capsules or the less strong tablets regularly as they cause constipation and could prevent the body absorbing other medication.

I am writing these words in early 2003 and can say that I have had no trouble for some months. I am aware that IBS is a recurring illness and could come back, so I am always alert to this possibility. As a safeguard, I carry prescribed capsules with me if I am to be away from home for any length of time. Although I am now back on a normal food routine, there are some adaptations I make all the time. Once I ate what many people would regard as an ultra-generous amount of fruit and vegetables. I now eat a slightly reduced amount and take great care to avoid skins. I am a great lover of nuts but eat them rarely and with caution. For some years I have curtailed consumption of wheat in any form to aid my arthritis, and I have discovered that wheat accentuates IBS in some cases. I am sure I have benefited by taking a daily probiotic and live yoghurt. Some of my favourite, and beneficial, dishes are the syllabubs on pages 184–5 and the smoothies on page 218. I particularly like the Autumn Special with its ginger flavour. Fortunately, I can make this any time of the year. I enjoy the dishes I have created from the recipes that follow. I do not feel I am being deprived of interesting meals at all.

Since IBS is so often allied to stress, I try to make my life as peaceful as possible, although I am still doing a considerable amount of work. There is no doubt that a condition such as IBS can cause one to panic. When I fear an attack may be coming on, I take the practical dietary steps given in this book. Also, no matter how busy I am, I take time out and spoil myself – and I think this is equally helpful. I listen to music, watch a light-hearted video or film or read a favourite book, preferably one that makes me laugh. I drink a delicious smoothie or cup of tea and enjoy something like a sweet biscuit or freshly baked scone. Tension eases; I am in control of my situation; I can cope with it; and sometimes I feel I may have averted an attack.

I know it is difficult to give up some of the foods you enjoy and replace them with new ones, but none of the recipes contains anything difficult to obtain or unpleasant. On the contrary, most of the ingredients are enjoyable. The dishes are simple to prepare, which is important, for neither you nor your carer will want to spend too long cooking. In following the help given in this book you should steadily begin to feel a wonderful sense of recovery and freedom from pain or discomfort.

I wish you good eating and renewed good health.

Marguerite Patten OBE

two the healthy gut

A healthy body depends on a healthy gut.

Marguerite Patten's story of her struggle with irritable bowel syndrome in Chapter 1 demonstrates dramatically the link between diet and the gut. The lesson from her experience is universal: some foods irritate and upset the gut, while others work to heal damaged tissues and restore normal digestive function. But which foods are which? Just what is the gut, and how does it work? *The Healthy Gut Cookbook* tackles these questions and explains how you can use choose the best foods to meet your digestive system's unique needs.

This chapter describes the structure of the gut and explains how its various parts perform different phases of the digestive process. To top things off, the liver – the largest and arguably most important organ in the body – is discussed and guidelines are given on how you can protect it.

Some people find the word *gut* disagreeable and perhaps a little coarse. In fact, it is a proper descriptive medical term and the title of a highly respected medical journal. In medical usage, *gut* refers to the small and large intestines, *gastrointestinal* describes the gut plus the stomach, and *digestive system* covers all parts of the body involved in the breakdown of food and absorption of nutrients, including the mouth, teeth, liver and pancreas. In this book, the three terms are used interchangeably.

It is not just words that make people feel uneasy; many of us find the need to describe the processes of the gut hugely embarrassing. Perhaps it is the influence of television chat shows and medical dramas, but talking about personal sexual or mental problems often comes easier than discussing the more awkward subject of digestion. Many older people find it rude to speak of 'fart' or 'faeces'. Fortunately, younger people seem less affected by these inhibitions. This text provides a balance of terms that will suit all. A later section suggests ways you can ask for help and accurately describe your symptoms with minimal embarrassment (*see page 228*).

how the gut controls your health

The gut is the gatekeeper between nutrients in the food we eat and the internal working of the body. When it is damaged by illness or injury, the inward flow of vital nutrients dwindles. The heart, muscles, blood and bones are denied the carbohydrates, proteins, vitamins and minerals needed for energy, repair and immunity. The healthiest diet, brimming with the finest foods, is useless to the body if all parts of the digestive system are not functioning in harmony.

STRUCTURE OF THE GUT

The gut is a hollow tube running through the body's core – top to bottom – from the mouth to the anus. Many writers compare it with a hole in a doughnut. This imagery suggests that the gut is an inert space, passively allowing the flow of food and drink from one end to the other. Nothing could be more misleading. The gut is a miraculous structure containing highly specialized parts capable of grinding, liquefying, extraction, absorption and elimination. Its cellular lining controls its many chemical processes, while its outer muscular wall kneads, moves and stores the material passing through it.

Modifications in the structure of the gut's lining are astounding. For example, the mouth has a smooth lining, but contains the tongue and teeth needed to chew and crush the food. In sharp contrast, the lining of the small intestine is deeply folded and covered with millions of tiny, finger-like protrusions call *villi*. The villi are packed with blood capillaries so close to their surface that proteins, sugars, fats and essential nutrients flow smoothly from the lumen of the gut into the bloodstream. Lower down the passageway, the digestive matter that remains after nutrients have been extracted comes in contact with friendly bacteria that bulk the mass. The walls of the gut remove excess water, and the remaining unwanted material (faeces) is stored before being expelled from the body. A problem anywhere along this chain of events can result in inefficiency or failure of the entire system. It is easy to see why the health of this low tube, with all its parts, determines how well your body functions and how well you feel.

The healthy gut is highly mobile, although we are usually unaware of its activity. Muscular contractions (*peristalsis*) mix and move food along the tube as digestion progresses. We are more aware of the gut's motility when things go wrong. For example, if contractions are slowed – by drugs, for example – constipation may be a result. Or, if their speed is increased due to stress, excessive amounts of caffeine, food poisoning or medication – a bout of diarrhoea may be in the offing.

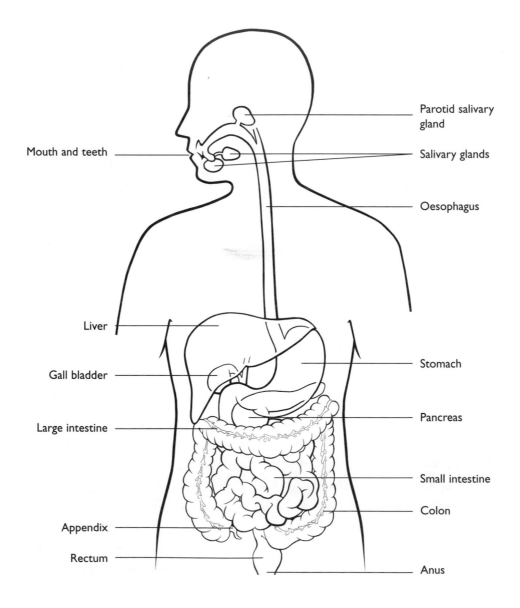

The major divisions of the digestive system are the *mouth, oesophagus, stomach, duodenum, small intestine, large intestine (colon), rectum* and *anus.* Along its path, several glands provide chemicals (enzymes) that aid the breakdown of certain food components: these are the salivary glands in the mouth, the pancreas and the gall bladder. Parts of the gut contain cells that secrete other chemicals needed for digestion. The stomach, for example, contains cells that secrete a strong acid.

In a healthy person, the contents from a meal take between 15 and 18 hours to pass from one end of the digestive tube to the other. Three to five hours are spent in the stomach, and about four hours in the small intestine where absorption of nutrients takes place.

Digestion begins in the *mouth,* where food is crushed and ground by the teeth and mixed with saliva containing enzymes that start breaking down starchy foods into simple sugars. Proper chewing is important. Food needs to be properly shredded to give maximum exposure to digestive enzymes, and saliva needs a chance to be mixed into the mass of food. After being swallowed, food is carried by muscular waves down the *oesophagus* and emptied into the stomach. A muscular valve (rather like a rubber band) prevents food and stomach fluid returning up the oesophagus.

The *stomach* is a large muscular pouch, or bulge, in the gut where food is thoroughly mixed and kneaded. Little is absorbed in the stomach other than certain drugs and alcohol. The lining in this part of the digestive tube contains two types of specialized cells: one secretes powerful hydrochloric acid needed to liquefy the food, and the other produces thick mucus needed to protect the lining of the stomach from its own acid. If the mucous barrier breaks down, ulcers can develop. Despite its acidic environment, the stomach can be infected with a bacterium, *Helicobacter pylori,* which is present in the majority of ulcer patients. (Ulcer treatment now includes antibiotics that eliminate this unwelcome intruder and speed healing.) From the stomach, the products of digestion pass through another rubber-band-like constriction (the *pyloric valve*) at the bottom of the stomach and enter the most important part of the digestive system: the small intestine.

The *small intestine* is about 7.5 metres (25 feet) in length and has three distinguishable parts: the *duodenum* (separated from the stomach by the pyloric valve), the *jejunum* and the *ileum.* Each is modified to perform a specific biochemical process. The first step must be to neutralize the digestive material coming from the stomach to make it slightly alkaline. This occurs in the duodenum, where bile manufactured by the liver and stored in the *gall bladder* joins alkaline fluids from the *pancreas* (needed to break down fats) and flows into the gut through a delicate structure called the *common bile duct.* (The pancreas also produces insulin needed to control blood sugar levels, but that hormone is transferred directly from the pancreas into the bloodstream.) By this time, the environment of the gut is watery. Pancreatic enzymes continue working as the digestive matter enters the jejunum, where enzymes produced by cells in the gut wall complete the breakdown of carbohydrates into sugars, fats into fatty acids and glycerol, and proteins into amino acids. Along the way vitamins, minerals and other compounds are released from the digested remains of food. The breakdown of food into its useful parts is called *digestion.*

Millions of finger-like *villi* rise out of the intestinal wall and are washed by the nutrient slurry passing through. Each is covered by a thin membrane of cells encasing a twist of blood capillaries so small that red blood cells flow through single file. Individual molecules of protein (*amino acids*), sugar, vitamins and minerals pass easily from the slurry into the bloodstream, which carries them to the liver for further processing within the body (*metabolism*). This passage is the normal case, and is called *absorption.* If villi are damaged by illness or poor diet, they tend to lie flat, thus hindering absorption. (Some fats are absorbed in a slightly different manner by the *lymphatic system*, a vast circulatory system of tiny tubes and glands involved in fighting infection and controlling fluid within the body.) By the time the food residue reaches the third part of the small intestine (ileum), it is fully digested. Nutrients are absorbed here, as are bile salts, which are returned to the liver. Unfortunately, toxic substances are also absorbed by the gut; these are passed to the liver for detoxification or storage.

Finally, the digested material reaches the large intestine (*colon, anus* and *rectum*). It enters the colon as a wet bulky mass consisting mainly of fibre (*see page 20 for information about fibre*). This part of the gut has modified villi that absorb water and leave the *faeces* or *stool* (bowel motion). But the colon contains something more: it contains millions – perhaps billions – of bacteria that help this final stage of digestion by breaking down fibre. (*More is said about gut bacteria under the section on Probiotics in the next chapter.*)

Like all other good 'systems', the digestive system is no better than any one of its parts. For example, at the start of the digestive tube, teeth are used to tear and crush food to facilitate its chemical breakdown in the stomach and gut. If food is not crushed and mixed properly – perhaps because of ill-fitting false teeth, or a rushed meal eaten under stress – the chemical processes that occur further along the tube will be less effective. If the chemical processes are less than effective, absorption of nutrients will be incomplete. When nutrients do not reach the body in quantities needed to keep tissues healthy because of a failure in the digestive process, a potentially dangerous condition called *malabsorption* occurs.

absorption and malabsorption

A fully functioning digestive system is needed to reap maximum benefit from a healthy diet. As noted above, the normal flow of nutrients from the gut into the body through the bloodstream is called absorption. When this process fails, malabsorption results. If malabsorption becomes severe, *malnutrition* sets in. Malnutrition destroys the body. It lowers resistance to infection, stunts physical and mental growth in children, causes infertility, and is to blame for the slow degeneration of bones, muscles and other organs. Many scientists believe that borderline nutritional deficiencies (in which the body receives smaller quantities of vital nutrients than are required by normal body functions) are at the root of heart disease, arthritis and possibly certain forms of cancer.

Symptoms of malabsorption are variable and may include weight loss, fatigue and foul-smelling, bulky diarrhoea. If untreated, malabsorption leads to illnesses as diverse as peripheral nerve damage and anaemia. Causes of malabsorption usually involve inflammation of the gut and include food sensitivities, Coeliac disease (*see page 58*), Crohn's disease (*see page 63*), chronic pancreatitis, advanced diabetes mellitus and cystic fibrosis. Left untreated, parasitic infection of the gut can also block the passage of nutrients.

There is evidence that a genetic factor contributes to the development of illnesses leading to malabsorption.

love your liver!

The largest organ in your body – the liver – deserves special attention. Protected by the ribs and tucked under the diaphragm, it contributes to the metabolism of fats and proteins, helps maintain normal blood sugar levels, is responsible for the formation and storage of energy as glycogen, and secretes bile to aid the digestion of fat. Of equal importance to its various roles in metabolism, the liver is the body's great detoxifier. It neutralizes alcohol, nicotine, drugs and poisons, and stores toxic substances that have no means of being excreted from the body. It is responsible for at least 22 chemical functions on which life depends.

You obviously need your liver, but how do you care for it? Unlike the muscular parts of the digestive system, which quickly let us know when something is wrong, the liver is a quiet organ that gives little trouble unless it has suffered serious damage. Here are some basic tips.

- Avoid recreational drugs!
- Avoid heavy drinking and excessive intake of spicy foods.
- Restrict intake of saturated fats from dairy products and fatty meats.
- Limit caffeinated drinks, such as coffee, tea and cola.
- Reduce your intake of refined sugar.
- Enjoy foods high in vitamin C. (Vitamin C may help the liver cope with detoxification, so enjoy strawberries, blackcurrants, green peppers, spinach and citrus fruit whenever possible.)
- Eat liver! It is a rich source of folic acid and vitamin B12. (These nutrients are needed for normal liver function. Other sources of folate include wheatgerm, nuts and green leafy vegetables. Vitamin B12 is found in lean red meat, eggs and fortified cereal.)
- Include oily fish in your diet at least once a week.
- Enjoy foods from plants, especially green leafy vegetables, artichokes and beetroot (see *Chapter 4*).

The liver regenerates itself to a certain extent, but will fail when overtaxed by alcohol or drug abuse, poor diet, infections or illnesses. Signs of chronic liver disease include yellowing of the whites of the eyes and skin (jaundice), loss of body hair, distended abdomen and fever.

three maintaining a healthy gut

 Few people blessed with a healthy gut know how to maintain and protect it. If the gut was a very expensive car, a fine camera – or even a top-of-the-line washing machine – we would take out the instruction book, read it from cover to cover, and make sure we followed the instructions to get the best possible service from our investment. The digestive system deserves the same care.

This chapter covers a range of topics that shed light on how to maintain a healthy gut, including how to eat, a modern approach to a balanced diet, and what you should look for on a yoghurt pot.

the pleasure of eating

How you eat your food helps determine whether or not you have a healthy gut.

Modern lifestyles – TV dinners, dependence on takeaway food, and a different social schedule for everyone in a household – work against healthy eating habits. We live in a rush-rush world where consuming food has become a necessity, rather than a source of pleasure and relaxation. Gulping down half-chewed food, overeating, washing everything down with fizzy drinks, and failing to relax during a meal can lead to indigestion, bloating and uncertain bowels. Can we doubt that bad eating habits contribute to the epidemic of gastric and bowel conditions plaguing most of Western society?

What is the basic rule of good gut health? *Meals should be eaten slowly at a table in a peaceful environment, taking time to enjoy both the food and the company of others.* This may seem simplistic, but the belief that how you eat is as important as what you eat has been taught for thousands of years. Wise men advised us not to think only about how we eat, but also how the food is prepared. The ancient Indian healing practice of Ayurveda tells us to prepare food while in a peaceful state of mind. It claims that the cook's mood enters the food, which in turn influences the mood of those who eat it. In other words, if you are tense and nervy when you poach the fish or season the Bolognese, those you feed will soon become tense and nervy, too.

There is some sense to this. Here is a case in point: sometimes Mum in the kitchen after a hard day's work is not a pretty sight. Perhaps the food she prepares is not really affected by her mood, but you can be sure that her exhaustion, or frustration, from a day in the office can charge the air with tension, destroying any chance of easy conversation and giving everyone at least a touch of indigestion! Food is a beautiful part of life. Enjoy cooking it and eating it. (*See the Glossary for more information about Ayurveda.*)

Adopting the Golden Rules of Eating, listed overleaf, is a good first step towards maintaining a healthier digestive system. Try applying this strategy to at least one meal each day. You can begin with breakfast, lunch or dinner – it does not matter. Over time, the 'practice' of relaxing during this one daily meal will help you develop healthier habits every time you eat. You might be pleasantly surprised by the speedy disappearance of belching, heartburn and flatulence you suffered in the past.

water – the foundation of life

If you want a healthy gut, drink an adequate amount of water.

Water is indispensable for life and makes up approximately 99 per cent of molecules within the cells of the human body. It is also essential for many processes in the body: watery amniotic fluid, for example, provides a safe surrounding for a growing foetus; transport of toxins and waste from the kidneys depends on water. And, more to the point here, a large part of digestion takes place in a watery environment. The internal messages that signal dehydration are clear – dry mouth, poor concentration and headaches. If we fail to respond to these signals the results can be constipation, the build-up of renal waste leading to kidney stones, and bladder infections when harmful

The golden rules of eating

⊙

1. Find at least a quarter of an hour to sit and relax before eating.
2. Do not over-burden your stomach with drinks and snack foods before mealtimes.
3. Always eat at a table using proper plates and cutlery. (No burgers from a bag or curries from disposable trays!)
4. Eat in pleasant surroundings. Enjoy calming music. A simple arrangement of flowers adds to a relaxed atmosphere.
5. Eat slowly, and chew food well before swallowing.
6. Keep conversation light; avoid discussing emotionally charged issues.
7. If you drink alcoholic beverages before or during a meal, do so in moderation.
8. After a main meal, go for a walk – after an unusually large meal, have a rest.

bacteria cannot be flushed away. Knowing these facts, many of us still fail to consume adequate amounts of water. Why is this so? Here are two common reasons:

- *Tap water is safe to drink but tastes unappealing.* If this sounds familiar, try adding a slice of fresh lemon to the glass before drinking. Simple charcoal filters remove both unpleasant tastes and most impurities. Chilled filtered tap water is a refreshing drink. Or, if finances allow, drink bottled water from a reputable source, or brand. (Some bottled water is little more than bottled tap water.)

- *Most public places have few, if any, safe places from which to drink.* When was the last time you saw a drinking fountain you would allow your children to use? As these are in such short supply you will probably need to get your water from a café or restaurant when you are out and about. Ask for water, even if you must pay for it, and don't be tempted to order a cup of coffee or fizzy drink instead. Milk or fresh fruit juice are healthy alternatives to water. If you resent paying for such a basic necessity, consider carrying a small bottle of water with you.

Some people rarely drink water, but keep their fluid intake topped up with tea, coffee, juices, fizzy drinks and alcoholic beverages. Is this a good idea? Remember that caffeine acts as a mild diuretic and may actually add to dehydration. Fizzy drinks contain artificial sweeteners, colours, flavours and preservatives with no nutritional value. Much of this extraneous material goes into the body to be detoxified and eliminated as waste, but some of it has an effect on our internal chemistry. For example, if you tend to suffer from headaches after 'a few too many', you are living proof that alcohol dehydrates the body.

GETTING ENOUGH WATER

The normal chemical processes within our body (metabolism) produce about a third of the total fluids we need, but what about the remainder? What we drink supplies about 60 per cent of our daily fluid intake, what we eat supplies the rest. It may surprise you to know that bread and cereals provide a source of water, and fruit and vegetables in a balanced diet can supply about 18 per cent of our needs. It is well to remember that eating plenty of soft fruit and vegetables provides water in addition to vitamins and minerals. If you are travelling and find yourself in a place where it may be difficult to get water, or where you do not trust the available drinking water, consider enjoying a freshly cut melon or a well-washed peach to quench your thirst.

It is difficult to say exactly how much water to consume because the body's requirements vary from person to person. Our level of activity and state of health influence our needs for water, as do environmental aspects like temperature and humidity. Obviously it is sensible to increase the fluid you drink if you have perspired heavily, or if the weather is hot and dry; but by how much? The answer varies according to both vogue and scientific opinion. The middle ground seems to be between four and six glasses (1½–1¾ litres/ 2½–3 pints) of water per day, with additional quantities drunk when needed to compensate for fluid lost through heavy exercise, weather and illness.

Like everything else in life, it is possible to get too much of a good thing: you actually do yourself harm by drinking too much water. Sports experts warn that some athletes – principally runners – put their health at risk in this way. Writing in the *Telegraph*, Peta Bee pointed out that, while hydration is important during sport, statements like 'you cannot drink too much water' and 'don't worry about the heat, just drink more' are wrong and dangerous. Water intoxication and other problems can occur that disrupt the body's salt balance, leading to dizziness, respiratory problems and even collapse. For those participating in strenuous exercise, such as long-distance running, a safe rule is to drink about half a glass (about a quarter of a pint) of water for every hour of exercise. Or, weigh yourself before and after exercise: replenish your fluid levels by drinking two medium glasses of water for every pound of weight lost.

fibre – a rough guide

- Build your meals around fruits and vegetables.
- Add foods high in complex carbohydrates (such as wholemeal pasta and bread, potatoes, rice, maize).
- Enjoy a single serving of high-protein foods (meat, eggs, dairy products, soya) at each meal.
- Top it off with a little of what you fancy. Unless you have a known medical condition that prohibits this luxury, a glass a wine or a small dish of ice cream will not break the nutritional bank.
- Cut down your intake of deep-fried and other fatty foods and refined carbohydrates (white bread and pasta, sugar), and limit your alcohol consumption. These foods are liabilities when it comes to good gut health.

Just like any other part of the body, a healthy gut requires a balanced intake of foods supplying the full complement of essential vitamins and minerals, proteins, carbohydrates and fats. In fact, the gut needs a more constant flow of nutrients than many other organ systems because the processes of digestion scour surface cells from the gut lining at an amazing rate: the lining of the gut is replaced every 72 hours. This rapid turnover increases its vulnerability to ulceration and inflammation.

What sets the nutritional needs of the gut apart is its need for fibre. This indigestible form of carbohydrate ferments in the gut with the help of local bacteria, and provides the bulk needed to push waste materials from the body. Fruits, vegetables, whole grains, nuts and seeds supply fibre, making them essential for a balanced diet. Most experts tell us that a balanced diet includes at least five portions of fruit and vegetables a day because these foods are rich sources of necessary nutrients, and because they are an excellent source of soluble fibre (the differences between soluble and insoluble fibre are discussed below).

The composition of a balanced diet is a hotly debated issue. As this book is being written the main excitement among slimmers concerns low-carbohydrate/high-protein diets; these appear to miraculously shift the body's chemistry so that unwanted fat melts away. This is an attractive idea seized upon by millions, but it has a drawback. Eating low-carbohydrate foods means restricting the consumption of fibre, and this can lead to the most common form of gut complaint: constipation. If you read Chapter 5, about diverticulitis and the various health problems involving constipation, you will see why this common condition should be avoided. There are ways to get around problems presented by low-carbohydrate diets. Laxatives are the most popular solution – but they can become habit forming and do not provide the benefit of minerals and vitamins found in a well-balanced diet.

High-protein diets are only one reason the problem of constipation is accelerating. The modern Western diet invites trouble by being based on foods that are low in fibre and high in refined sugar and saturated fats – all of which are bad for the gut. As a result, every day more of us are afflicted by indigestion, gastric ulcers, flatulence, diverticulitis and constipation, leading to serious bowel disease, including cancer. Both soluble and insoluble fibre help reduce this risk. Eating brown rice, bran and nuts provides insoluble fibre. Fresh fruits and vegetables, brown bread, oats and pulses are rich sources of soluble fibre. Dried fruits and whole grains provide both. When planning a balanced diet, include sources of both types of fibre.

There are significant differences in the two types of fibre. Insoluble fibre has no known health benefit other than providing bulk to discourage constipation. Like the soluble form, it consists of complex and indigestible carbohydrates. To a limited extent, insoluble fibre helps sustain the normal bacterial flora of the gut, which also add to the weight and bulk of the waste – or stool – as it works its way through the lower bowel. Without bulk, the muscular walls of the intestine get flabby and relaxed, and fail to be efficient.

Soluble fibre, on the other hand, gives up its form and dissolves in the watery environment of the digestive system. Consider what happens when you prepare porridge. As the oats cook and pieces of grain swell, the simmering water or milk begins to thicken and become viscous due to the release of soluble fibre. In the gut, the same molecules that thicken the porridge can absorb various substances (such as bile) during digestion, preventing their transfer into the bloodstream. Considerable research evidence suggests that this nutritionally inert substance not only supports good gut health, but also helps reduce blood cholesterol levels and prevents sharp fluctuations in blood sugar.

food and cancer

The right foods help prevent cancer. In 1997, a major research report by the World Cancer Research Fund, *Food, Nutrition and the Prevention of Cancer*, announced that what you eat dramatically affects your cancer risk. One recommendation stands out from all others: individuals can significantly decrease their risk of developing certain cancers by increasing their intake of fruits and vegetables. Based on this report, the British food writer Oliver Gillie produced *Food for Life, Preventing Cancer through Healthy Diet* in 1998. His advice is:

- *Enjoy a plant-based diet rich in its variety of fruits, vegetables and pulses. Minimize your intake of starchy staple foods.*
- *Eat 400–800 grams (15–30 ounces) of fruits and non-root or tuberous vegetables a day – every day of the year (this works out to be five or more servings).*
- *Eat 600–800 grams (20–30 ounces) of mixed cereals and root or tuberous vegetables and plantains.*
- *Choose minimally processed foods and restrict consumption of refined sugar.*
- *If meat is your source of protein, give it a low priority; 80 grams (3 ounces) a day is adequate for adults. Preferred meats are fish, poultry and meat from non-domesticated animals (venison and hare from reputable sources are excellent foods).*
- *Limit your intake of saturated fat. (Fat is part of a healthy diet. Tip your fat intake towards unsaturated fats like those in oils, nuts, olives and avocados.)*
- *Alcohol is 'not recommended'. (Keep your intake well within safe limits. See pages 27–8.)*
- *Avoid charred foods. (Skip the blackened barbecued steak, especially the charred fat.)*
- *Limit your salt intake and avoid salted and preserved foods.*

Since publication of the report by the World Cancer Research Fund, medical and governmental authorities have flooded the news media with information about the importance of eating fruit and vegetables; five portions a day has been recommended as a healthy dietary goal for everyone. There is scant evidence, however, that the general public has taken the message on board. Women, and particularly younger women, appear to be more receptive to the message than other demographic groups, but most men still look upon fruit and vegetables as uninteresting food. Of even greater concern, recent studies of children's diets show they fall far short of ideal.

probiotics

In her personal story, Marguerite Patten writes about her experience with irritable bowel syndrome. Like many others suffering from serious illnesses of the digestive system, probiotics helped her regain control over her body and maintain good health. We see references to probiotics in the health media, and new lines of probiotic foods and supplements appear in the shops almost monthly. But questions still remain: what are probiotics; how do they work; and what do they have to do with food? The answers are all about bacteria.

According to Lennart Cedgårt, MD, writing for www.positivehealth.com, *dysbiosis* is a major cause of intestinal illness ('dys' means faulty, and 'bios' means life and growth). Put simply, the faulty growth of gut bacteria causes problems. 'Pro' biosis is needed to correct faulty bacterial growth and support a healthy environment within the gut.

The presence of bacteria in the intestines was mentioned in Chapter 2. These organisms contribute to the absorption of minerals, proteins and vitamins from the gut; they break down (ferment) fibrous food residue and combine with water and digestive sludge to form the bulk (stool or faeces) eventually evacuated from the body. Different types of bacteria live and multiply in the gut. Under normal conditions they exist in a happy balance, but this can be altered radically by stress, medication, eating tainted food and a poor diet.

Sometimes the mere introduction of a new strain of healthy bacteria can cause a major upset, something experienced by many travellers. After the first day in a foreign location there may be a noticeable change in the gut, perhaps signalled by rumbling and flatulence, and sometimes something more extreme. A day later, the problem is gone. Food eaten can came from the best and cleanest hotels and restaurants, but the problem is difficult to avoid. While you are enjoying the tastes and textures of delicious new foods, your stomach is encountering a new strain of one or more of the normal bacteria inhabiting your gut. It takes time for things to adjust. Here are two pieces of good advice: go easy on food and drink for the first 24 hours after you arrive at your destination, and always carry lactic bacteria (probiotics) supplements with you. Starting probiotics before your arrival can minimize the risk of feeling unwell.

Probiotics contain healthy (lactic) bacteria known to convert sugars into lactic acid. This action is important in the human gut, and in the fermentation of foods such as yoghurt, cheese and buttermilk. You can add lactic bacteria to your digestive system either by including 'live' yoghurt in your diet at least once a day, or by taking a commercial supplement. Live yoghurt (which has not been treated or processed in a way that kills bacteria) is a good choice because it is rich in calcium and adds real flavour to food. Many of Marguerite Patten's recipes for smoothies and tempting dishes include yoghurt for these reasons. Well-known lactic bacteria you may see listed on a food label are: *Lactobacillus acidophilus, L. bulgaricus, Streptococcus thermophilus* and *Bifido bacterium bifidum.*

During the process of breaking down fibre in the lower gut, lactic bacteria produce an acidic environment harmful to bacteria that survive in alkaline conditions. This is the primary contribution lactic bacteria make, although most strains also fight dangerous bacteria by producing a specific form of antibiotic: *L. bulgaricus* produces bulgarican, for example.

The balance of friendly lactic bacteria in the gut can be disrupted by the contraceptive pill, steroids and antibiotics: taking probiotics helps put things right. A few hours after taking a dose of antibiotics, take a probiotics supplement (or eat live yoghurt) to avoid destruction of healthy gut bacteria. Other conditions of the gut known to respond to probiotics include gastric ulcers, infectious diarrhoea, constipation, indigestion, Crohn's disease, ulcerative colitis, irritable bowel syndrome and irritable bowel disease. Writing in the *Journal of the Royal Society of Medicine* (April 2003), doctors Daisy Jonkers and Reinhold Stockbrügger of the Netherlands reviewed the medical literature for research into the use of probiotics. They concluded that the evidence is promising, with encouraging results reported even in such complex conditions as irritable bowel disease (colitis and Crohn's disease).

food combining

Many nutritional therapists advise certain clients to avoid eating carbohydrate foods and protein foods at the same meal. This approach to diet (food combining) is commonly known as the Hay diet, after Dr Hay, who first publicized the possible benefits of this practice. The theory is that eating both proteins and carbohydrates at the same meal hinders digestion. Most medical experts are dubious, but many people suffering from gastric ailments find food combining works for them.

There are good reasons to believe it has benefits, especially in cases where the digestive system is weakened by illness (e.g. ulcers), medication (e.g. NSAIDs; *see page 70*), or injury (e.g. alcohol poisoning). Proteins and carbohydrates are digested in very different ways and require contrasting digestive environments. Proteins, for example, stimulate the production of highly acidic gastric juices in the stomach, while carbohydrates are digested in neutral-to-slightly-alkaline conditions further along the digestive tube, in the intestines. A normal, healthy gut can simultaneously deal with both; that is how most of us eat. But if the system is flagging, the digestive processes may be affected. One theory suggests that excessive acids produced in the stomach during the digestion of protein may be difficult to neutralize, thus slowing the breakdown of carbohydrates.

The well-respected American nutritional therapist, Paul Pitchford, takes a comprehensive approach to food combining in his book, *Healing with Whole Foods*. He presents three different eating plans. The first (Plan A) is designed to improve normal digestion, and is based on four rules:

1   Proteins are eaten early in a meal, followed by carbohydrates. For example, meaty antipasti before pasta with herbs and garlic, followed by fruit. Remember: simpler meals digest better.
2   Salty foods should be eaten first.
3   Proteins should be combined with non-starchy green vegetables.
4   Sweet foods and fruit should be eaten alone or in small quantities at the end of the meal.

Plan B is for people with sensitive digestive systems or who are ill. The basic rules are the same as for Plan A, but in this case proteins and carbohydrates must be separated into different meals, with green non-starchy vegetables eaten with both. Tomatoes, lemon and the juice of limes can be combined with meat because they add to the acidity during digestion. (This makes a small steak served with a lettuce and tomato salad, dressed with olive oil and lemon juice, a healthy meal – if you skip the chips!) Fruits are to be eaten alone. Milk and dairy products are not to be combined with meat.

The third Pitchford plan for food combining is a surprise. Plan C champions the 'one pot meal', which echoes traditional cooking in India, China and other parts of the world. No attempt is made to separate foods: they all go in a pot with plenty of water and are allowed to cook together slowly over a low heat where a kind of pre-digestion takes place. One expert in this kind of cooking is quoted as saying, 'The various foods have settled their differences in the pot.' These are watery foods – stews, soups and congees – and ideal for people who are weak, chronically ill or who have trouble chewing. They are also good for the rest of us. A home-made soup or stew is a real treat when you are tired and cold. This is old-fashioned comfort food at its best!

the BRAT diet: bananas, rice, apples and toast

A bad case of diarrhoea and vomiting can lead to the body becoming dehydrated. These symptoms of bacterial infection rob the body of fluid and minerals needed to survive. It is essential that the fluid loss is reversed (rehydration) as quickly as possible. Only a few decades ago, people, especially the very young, died from dehydration caused by gastric illness. This changed when a cheap, fast and easy means of reversing fluid and mineral loss was discovered: a simple mix of table salt and sugar in clean water.

It is just as likely that you will experience fluid and mineral loss due to stomach illness at home as in some remote part of the world. Rehydration mixes will help (*see page 84*), but that is only part of the answer. You will also want to get your gut back to normal. A few years ago, a research team at Harvard University devised a simple diet that gently restores the body's fluid balance and digestive processes. Based on bananas, rice, apples and toast, it is called the BRAT diet, and is highly recommended for all those who want a safe way to restore normal function to an ailing gut.

Remember: you may feel better soon after a bout of 'stomach flu', but it takes time for the delicate tissues of the intestine to regenerate.

THE BRAT PRINCIPLES

- *During the course of severe vomiting and/or diarrhoea, sip a rehydration mix (see page 84). As you feel better, slowly increase your fluid intake.*
- *About 24 hours after the last bout of illness, begin eating small amounts of foods from the following list. Increase your intake over a 24-hour period.*
- Bananas *provide energy and potassium, a mineral essential for your body to maintain a normal fluid balance. Potassium loss results in muscle weakness, mental confusion and – in extreme cases – heart problems.*
- Rice and toast *both provide low-fibre carbohydrates unlikely to irritate the bowel. Your first one or two pieces of toast should be dry, but then you can add a thin layer of butter or sweet spread, such as honey, depending on how you feel.*
- Apples *are believed to clean the digestive system. They are particularly helpful if your fluid loss was due to diarrhoea. Grated raw apples or cooked apples will do.*
- *After about 48 hours you can supplement this diet with a little boiled potato (skip the butter), cooked eggs and boiled vegetables, such as carrots. If these are tolerated well, slowly return to your normal diet.*

The BRAT diet may work wonders, but it can also be depressingly dull. Marguerite Patten has devised a variety of practical, tasty and easy-to-eat dishes based on these foods. They are delicious any time, but particularly when you are not feeling well.

what not to eat and drink

Alcohol and certain foods wreak havoc on the stomach and digestive system if taken in excess. If you plan to maintain a healthy gut, here is the bald truth about how we should temper our intake of food and drink!

- *Alcoholic beverages – men should limit themselves to 21 units per week; women should consume no more that 14. That translates into 3 and 2 units per day respectively. Avoid binge drinking – your stomach may rebel, but your liver will suffer in silence until it is too late. Each of the following is a single unit:*

- *Spirits: single pub measure = 25ml*
- *Fortified wine: single pub measure = 50ml*
- *Wine: single pub measure = 125ml*
- *Ordinary beer or lager (3.5%): small can = 275ml*
- *Strong beer or lager (7%): ½ small can = 135ml*

- *Avoid foods that are too hot (temperature).*
- *Go easy on foods containing excessive quantities of hot peppers.*
- *Limit your caffeine intake. Experts suggest not drinking more than six caffeinated beverages a day (tea, coffee, cola). Drink less if you suffer from stomach ulcers, kidney disease, heart problems or high blood pressure. Caffeine is a mild stimulant commonly used to improve alertness and mental performance. Used in excess it causes insomnia, loss of calcium from bone, palpitations and tremors. In some people it triggers joint inflammation and migraines. Caffeine is addictive and can cause unpleasant withdrawal symptoms such as severe headaches and irritability.*

lifestyle and the gut

If you want a healthy gut, live a healthy life!

How can we be surprised that diseases of the gut are on the increase when we know that our modern Western lifestyle is often less than healthy? Too much fat around the middle, smoking and lack of exercise set the stage for an unhealthy gut. Other habits that contribute towards gut problems are drinking excessive amounts of alcohol, using recreational drugs, running on the ragged edge of mental and physical exhaustion, caffeine addiction and consuming fatty takeaway foods as standard fare. Specific facts about how these lifestyle choices affect the gut are discussed in Chapter 5, 'When Things Go Wrong'. Hundreds of self-help books and videos are available to help you overcome your personal lifestyle problems.

the ageing gut

Passing years affect the way we look and feel. Our skin changes, we tend to feel less energetic, and we suffer more from niggling aches and pains due to wear and tear on joints and muscles. To fight off the years, we may try a new face cream, join a gym or start a diet designed to correct whatever we feel affects us most. We worry about our hearts, our brains, our muscles and our bones. And yet, as strange as it may seem, very few of us stop to worry about our ageing digestive system. We fail to recognize that caring for this part of our body can not only improve the way we feel, but – best of all – increase the likelihood we will live longer, healthier lives. Here are just a few ways ageing – and our behaviour as we age – affects our digestive system.

- *Lost teeth and poorly fitted dentures can interfere with chewing. This makes it less likely that food will be crushed and mixed before reaching the stomach, thus slowing digestion.*
- *Many people avoid fresh fruits, such as apples, and nuts because they are hard to chew, missing out on needed vitamins, minerals and fibre.*
- *Meat may become difficult to chew – or prepare – and appears less frequently on the table, potentially reducing the intake of protein and vitamin B12 below healthy limits.*
- *Older people tend to drink too little water, thus failing to provide the watery environment needed for digestion. (Those worried about bladder control frequently suffer from this problem.)*
- *The stomach produces less acid with age, reducing the ability to digest proteins.*
- *Fewer digestive enzymes and secretions are produced by the pancreas and gut.*
- *Health problems may increase the need for regular medication that may have side-effects, altering the gut (see Appendix Two).*
- *A poor appetite and decreased activity are associated with ageing. A lowered food intake means that the body has less chance of getting the nutrients it needs.*
- *Smoking and drinking alcohol are habits that may become stronger with age. Smoking is sure to damage health. Consumed beyond moderation, alcohol can impair mental and physical health.*
- *Many older people may suffer from low levels of vitamin D because they tend to stay indoors, thus getting little exposure to sunlight.*
- *Preparing food becomes a bother and there is greater reliance on ready meals, thus reducing the intake of fresh fruit and vegetables.*

All these factors lead to poor nutrition. Scientific studies have shown that it is not uncommon for older people to consume less than their daily requirement of calcium, magnesium, zinc, folate, and vitamins B6, B12 and D. There is only one word to describe the consequences: *malnutrition*! The cost is high. Consider one fact: low levels of just one of the nutrients listed, vitamin B12, can lead to poor balance and coordination and memory lapses.

What can be done about this? The simple basics are:

- *Stay physically active to work up a good appetite.*
- *Make an effort to eat fresh foods that are a natural source of the nutrients you need.*
- *Find a pleasant place to sit in the sun and let your body build up valuable levels of vitamin D, the sunshine vitamin.*
- *Drink plenty of water.*
- *Choose simple-to-digest forms of protein, such as meaty soups and consommés.*
- *Enjoy live yoghurt whenever possible, and eat fresh fruits and vegetables every day.*

If you feel that this is not enough, talk to your local chemist or doctor about taking vitamin supplements. If you wear dentures, see your dentist and make certain they fit properly. Later chapters explain how choosing the right foods can help you maintain a healthy body – no matter what your age!

Remember: Medical evidence shows that older people who eat plenty of fruits and vegetables live longer, healthier lives.

food allergies, intolerances and sensitivities

Not everything on your plate may be good for you. Eating the wrong foods can cause a variety of symptoms ranging in severity from mild headaches and constipation to life-threatening anaphylactic shock. Other symptoms are hives, skin rash, asthma and inflammation of the bowel. There is no agreement on how reactions to food should be classified, but in general, any reaction causing asthma, hives, swelling and potentially fatal anaphylactic shock is a *food allergy*. Migraine, nausea, gastro-intestinal distress and wind are most frequently referred to as symptoms of *food intolerances*. Less well-defined symptoms occurring when a food, or member of a group of foods, is consumed may be classified as *food sensitivities*.

FOOD ALLERGIES

Food allergies arise when a normal food acts as an antigen or foreign substance in the body, setting off a train of events in the immune system leading to the release of antibodies. Allergies cause severe symptoms arising anywhere in the body. A typical scenario would be a woman enjoying crabmeat salad for lunch. Suddenly she experiences tingling lips, then swelling of the mouth and tongue, followed swiftly by a severe asthma attack.

FOOD INTOLERANCES

Food intolerances are diagnosed when antibodies to an allergen cannot be found. Unfortunately, some medical personnel tend to dismiss the idea of food intolerances because there is no clear-cut allergic response. These conditions may have less dire consequences, but nonetheless can cause real illness. Two examples of food intolerances are *gluten intolerance* (see Crohn's disease, *page 63*), where the body reacts to gluten in wheat, rye and barley, and *lactose intolerance*, where the body reacts to substances in cow's milk. Why people become sensitive to gluten is not clear, but we do know that lactose intolerance develops when the body is deficient in an enzyme needed to digest milk and milk products. This is not an 'allergic' reaction but a failure of the body's biochemistry. Lactose intolerance can cause belching and flatulence, either constipation or diarrhoea, and catarrh. A recurring crackly cough with no sign of infection may indicate a milk intolerance! In babies, symptoms of milk intolerance include chronic blocking of the nose (rhinitis), glue ear, colic and asthma. People changing from a diet containing little or no dairy products may find they develop lactose intolerance when they begin eating substantial amounts of milk and cheese. In these cases, the condition rights itself as the body begins producing the necessary digestive enzymes.

FOOD SENSITIVITIES

Food sensitivities are more difficult to define, and some doctors cast doubt on their existence. Most often, your own body is the best judge of what makes you unwell. If symptoms persist, an elimination diet will help. Elimination diets vary, but in all cases foods are either withdrawn or introduced into the diet under a prescribed eating programme. Undertaking this diagnostic procedure on your own is possible, but help from a professional nutritional therapist or dietitian will provide a comprehensive and objective view of your problem. A list of helpful addresses and websites is found at the back of this book.

Foods most frequently linked with food allergies and intolerances are:

Eggs may cause stomach upset, asthma and eczema.

Avoid egg white and all foods made with eggs, including baked goods, ice cream and mayonnaise.

Fish may cause digestive upset, rash and migraine.

Avoid all smoked fish and fish pâté; check to see if you are sensitive to white fish, such as cod and haddock.

Food additives may cause hyperactivity, migraines, flatulence and indigestion.

Avoid food and drink containing additives; watch out for benzoic acid, tartrazine and monosodium glutamate.

Gluten can cause migraine and coeliac disease (Crohn's disease).

Avoid wheat, rye and barley, and products made from these grains. Gluten is used as an additive by the food industry to improve the appearance and texture of many products. Unless specifically stated to the contrary, assume that all stock cubes contain gluten.

Milk (cow's) and products made with cow's milk can cause gastric upset, constipation, catarrh, eczema and wind.

Avoid cow's milk products. Ewe's milk and goat's milk are less likely to cause problems. Soya milk is another alternative, although some people find it causes indigestion.

Nuts can cause rash, eczema, swelling, asthma, and death due to anaphylactic shock.

Avoid all nuts and products containing nuts. Most food manufacturers are becoming conscious of this problem and labelling foods that may pose a danger. ALWAYS READ THE LABEL ON THE PACKAGE. Restaurants are more difficult; if you are concerned, call ahead to check how the chef deals with cases of nut allergy.

Shellfish can cause rash, nausea, stomach upset, asthma and death due to anaphylactic shock.

Avoid shellfish and all products containing shellfish. Watch out for fish soups and mixed fish salads, as they may contain shellfish or shellfish stock.

four good foods for a healthy gut

And when you crush an apple with your teeth, say to it in your heart,
'Your seeds shall live in my body,
And the buds of your tomorrow shall blossom in my heart,
And your fragrances shall be my breath,
And together we shall rejoice through all the seasons.'

KHALIL GIBRAN, *THE PROPHET*

This chapter is about foods that benefit the gut. Information has been gathered from three different healing systems: modern medicine, traditional Chinese medicine, and the ancient Indian practices of Ayurveda (*read more about these healing methods in the Glossary*). The extent of overlap between these healing systems is remarkable: all three recognize the health benefits of garlic and ginger, for example. With a few exceptions, these healing foods are fruits and vegetables. Meat, fish and fowl are mostly excluded, not because they are unimportant, but because of a simple truth: **the vast majority of nature's therapeutic substances are found in plants**.

We all know that nuts, seeds, root vegetables, fruits, leafy vegetables – and even flowers – provide vitamins, minerals and other nutrients needed for human development, health and reproduction. But that is not all. Beneficial parts of plants are as basic as the structural fibre in fruits and root vegetables, and as complex as molecules responsible for the colour of a flower or the content of a seed. Scientific research exploring the properties of plant compounds has already unearthed the therapeutic potential of isoflavones, indoles and lycopene, and more information will come. Research is important, but in many cases it only elaborates on what we already know: certain foods have specific benefits.

The following list of healthy gut foods will help you select ingredients and prepare meals that meet your unique digestive requirements. If, for example, you tend to develop constipation, try substituting yams or sweet potatoes for white potatoes once or twice a week. If you suffer from frequent intestinal infections, try selecting fruits and vegetables rich in natural antibacterial substances: garlic, onions, blackcurrants and apples are ideal choices. Build these foods into your personal plan to eat five or more servings of fruits and vegetables per day.

A 'serving' of fruits or vegetables is as follows:

- ¼ cup dried fruit
- 1 piece of fruit, ½ cup diced fruit, ½ cup fresh berries or grapes
- 1 cup 100% fruit juice (not fruit extracts or concentrates)
- 1 cup raw leafy vegetable (lettuce, spinach, bok choy, endive)
- ½ cup cooked vegetables, such as carrots and beets, and cooked green vegetables, such as beans and spinach
- ½ cup onions, leeks or spring onions (may be a combination of all alliums)
- 2 cloves garlic
- ½ cup cooked pulses (lentils, chickpeas, beans)
- ½ cup cooked grain (rice, bulgar, buckwheat, oats, barley)
- ½ cup grated raw carrots (most other raw root vegetables can be hard to digest)

In the following chapter, 'When Things Go Wrong', you will learn which foods to enjoy and which to avoid in the case of 20 different digestive disorders, and two or more of Marguerite Patten's healthy-gut recipes are recommended for each. Remember: adapting your diet can help control both the symptoms of illness and the side-effects of medication.

Use foods sensibly. Do not 'overdose' on specific items. When eaten in large quantities, many foods — figs and turmeric, for example — can upset your system. Remember that many herbs and spices contain powerful substances and all should be eaten in moderation.

healthy gut foods

ALLIUM (GARLIC, ONION, SHALLOTS, LEEKS)

If you are susceptible to gut infections (gastroenteritis), or are heading for a holiday destination where food preparation may be a bit haphazard, choose foods rich in these vegetables. They may have a 'pong', but they contain antibacterial, antiviral and antifungal compounds that help prevent infection. The same advice applies to anyone with a weakened immune system, or who has been taking antibiotics.

Counter the unpleasant breath odour by topping foods with lots of chopped parsley, or try chewing caraway seeds.

Research has shown these vegetables to be useful in preventing heart disease, and they may play a role in preventing cancer.

ALLSPICE

A spice used to aid digestion, this is a favourite flavour in several cuisines.

ALMOND OIL

When used in modest quantities (a teaspoonful per serving), this soothing oil can help calm gastric pain. If you find it unpleasant to take on its own, try blending it in a salad dressing, or use in a sauce for fish.

ALMONDS

Eating almonds is obviously an excellent way to consume almond oil in its most natural form; they are also highly nutritious and contribute to a healthy diet. A word of warning: remove the skins from the almond kernel before eating. According to the ancient Indian healing tradition of Ayurveda, the skin of the almond can irritate the stomach lining, and should not be eaten.

The oil in ground almonds can become rancid with time; use freshly ground nuts.

APPLES

It makes me want to call out – 'Is there an apple in the house?'
C.A. LEJEUNE

Ancient healers valued apples as one of nature's most healing foods. Today, scientific research suggests they contain a high level of natural antibiotics. Apples are an excellent source of soluble fibre, vitamin C and bioflavonoids. Peeled, grated and raw, apples are an old and trusted treatment for constipation. Stewed, they are useful in the treatment of gastritis and diarrhoea. Apples can be used as healing foods for people suffering from colitis and diverticulitis. Paul Pitchford, an internationally respected nutritional therapist, claims that apples and their juice benefit the liver and gall bladder, and actually soften gallstones.

Flavour apple sauce with healing spices, such as cinnamon, cardamom and nutmeg, to aid digestion and calm flatulence.

Remember: always wash apples well so you can enjoy eating the peel.

APRICOTS (DRIED)

Apricots are rich in nutrients including iron, copper, cobalt, potassium and betacarotene. They are an ideal ingredient when cooking for people suffering from gastric ulcers and/or mouth ulcers. A high fibre content makes apricots a useful choice when you are trying to avoid constipation, especially when you are pregnant or taking medications known to cause this problem.

ARTICHOKES (GLOBE)

The secret substance in these delicious flower heads is cynarin, which is thought to promote the flow of bile and aid the digestion of fats. Artichokes are used as a healing food in cases of gallstones and liver disease.

Artichokes are thought to settle the lower bowel and help control flatulence, thus aiding the management of irritable bowel syndrome.

Scientific evidence suggests that artichokes may help control blood cholesterol levels.

Remember: globe artichokes and Jerusalem artichokes are not related to one another, and only the former contains these health benefits. Jerusalem artichokes are root vegetables known for causing flatulence.

AVOCADOS

Ripe avocados can be used as a healing food in cases of stomach ulcers. A mild and nutritious fruit, they are a delicious and highly digestible source of the omega-6 essential fatty acid, linoleic acid. Some nutritionists believe these delicious fruits also contain a substance that helps eliminate uric acid from the body.

Avocados are an ideal food for people who have lost weight through illness, but do not want to increase their saturated fat intake by eating red meat and dairy foods.

BANANAS

One of the great natural foods, bananas are most easily digested in their ripe state. Packed with nutrients, they are an excellent choice for ulcer patients because there is evidence they stimulate the production of mucus in the gut, protecting the stomach from its own outpouring of gastric acid.

Remember: unripe bananas can cause flatulence. Bananas have been known to occasionally trigger migraines.

See 'The BRAT Diet', page 26.

BARLEY

Barley water is a drink known to aid the pain of constipation and cystitis. Easy to digest, the grain has a soothing effect on an inflamed gut, unless the cause is coeliac disease or gluten intolerance (*see page 58*). Traditional Chinese medicine tells us that barley helps regulate digestion and strengthen the pancreas.

BASIL

Used to aid stomach cramps and relieve nausea, this popular herb is said to calm the nervous system.

BEETROOT

Thought to be useful in detoxification of the liver, beetroot is beneficial to the entire digestive system. Drinking beetroot juice (or beetroot in a smoothie) may increase the flow of bile and aid the digestion of fats. Be aware that beetroot can cause false bleeding (*see the Glossary*).

BERRIES (GENERAL) AND RED GRAPES

Dark-skinned berries and grapes contain natural antibacterial substances that may benefit cases of colitis, diverticulitis, gastric ulcers and gastroenteritis. People with lowered immune systems should include these fruits in their diet at least once a day to help ward off infection. Enjoying these fruits as part of your normal diet helps maintain a healthy gut.

BILBERRIES

These plump blue fruits are a rich source of natural antibacterial compounds useful in combating gut infections. They are also rich in vitamin C and other substances that support the immune system.

BLACK PEPPER

An excellent aid to digestion, this highly valued spice also relieves constipation and eases flatulence.

BLACKCURRANTS

Rich in antibacterial substances known as anthocyanins, which inhibit dangerous forms of *E. Coli*, this fruit helps combat infections.

BLUEBERRIES

In traditional medicine these berries were dried and used to treat diarrhoea caused by food poisoning. Modern scientific investigation suggests that they contain compounds called anthocyanins, which are the source of this healing power.

Blueberries also contain a natural diuretic that helps clean the kidneys.

BRAN

Oat, rice and wheat bran can help prevent constipation, piles (haemorrhoids), diverticulitis and bowel cancer because it adds fibre, or bulk, to the diet and aids the normal passage of waste from the digestive system.

If you suffer from sensitivity to gluten, or have Crohn's disease, only use rice bran.

Use bran in moderation. Too much will cause bloating and may increase the symptoms of irritable bowel syndrome.

As an added benefit, the soluble fibre in oat bran is thought to reduce blood cholesterol levels and aid people with diabetes by improving sugar metabolism.

BROCCOLI

A rich source of vitamin C and other nutrients that promote good gut health, broccoli also contains compounds which scientists believe help prevent gastric and other cancers.

BUCKWHEAT

Traditional medicine claims buckwheat is useful in treating chronic diarrhoea, strengthening the digestive system and improving the appetite.

A good source of fibre, buckwheat helps prevent constipation and complications related to it. Free of gluten, buckwheat is an excellent choice of carbohydrate for those who suffer from wheat intolerance or Crohn's disease.

High in rutin (a substance shown to strengthen the walls of capillaries, like those found in the villi of the small intestine), buckwheat helps maintain the part of the digestive system responsible for normal absorption of nutrients. For more information about the structure of the digestive system, see pages 9–13.

CABBAGE

Including this somewhat maligned vegetable in your diet can help heal stomach ulcers. Scientific evidence suggests that S-Methylmethionine and other substances in cabbage promote the healing of gastric ulcers by stimulating the production of mucus to protect the stomach lining. Like other members of the brassica family (broccoli, cauliflower, kale and Brussels sprouts), cabbage is thought to help prevent gastric cancer.

Remember: eaten in excess, cabbage may cause wind and – in extreme cases – can cause iron deficiency and thyroid problems.

CAMOMILE

Tea made from the daisy-like flowers of this plant calms the nervous and digestive systems and helps relieve stress. Its healing properties are useful in controlling heartburn, gastritis and diverticulitis. Reach for camomile if you want a good comfort drink on those nights when you cannot sleep.

CARAWAY

Used as a spice in cuisines from Asia to Scandinavia, the tasty seeds of this plant stimulate the appetite and help relieve heartburn, wind and colic.

CARDAMOM

Another international favourite, this spice relieves heartburn, belching, excess stomach acid, wind and vomiting. Its healing properties are useful in the treatment of IBS. When chewed, cardamom seeds sweeten the breath.

CARROTS

High in natural sugars, fibre and betacarotene, these root vegetables help prevent constipation and provide nutrients needed to maintain a healthy gut.

Cooking releases nutrients from this fibrous vegetable, giving carrot purée an edge over carrot sticks. Peel carrots unless they are organic.

CELERY

The stalks and seeds of celery contain anti-inflammatory substances, which have been shown to aid the treatment of stomach ulcers and bowel inflammation. Celery is thought to benefit the liver and stimulate digestion. Research suggests celery helps lower blood cholesterol.

CHEDDAR CHEESE

This favourite British cheese contains substances considered to be useful in the treatment of gastric ulcers.

CHERRIES

The mild laxative effect of this fruit helps prevent and relieve constipation. Cherries are thought to contain natural substances that cleanse the system and help control gout. They are a good source of potassium, needed for energy and fluid balance.

CHERVIL

A herb that stimulates digestion, chervil is also known to ease the pain of heartburn.

CHICORY

Often used in the detoxification of the liver. Wild chicory is more effective than cultivated varieties.

CHILLI PEPPERS

Used in excess, chilli peppers may cause gastric irritation. However, when consumed in moderation they help control inflammation, provide vitamin C, and help relieve sinus congestion that may cause bad breath. Perhaps surprisingly, they are sometimes used in small amounts to relieve indigestion.

CHIVES

A member of the allium family (*see page 35*), chives stimulate the appetite and help digestion during convalescence.

CINNAMON

Useful in the treatment of diarrhoea, indigestion and wind, this popular spice also helps prevent bad breath by cleaning the sinuses.

CITRUS FRUIT (INCLUDING LEMONS, ORANGES, GRAPEFRUIT AND LIMES)

Grapefruit benefits the gut by stimulating digestion and alleviating belching.

Lemons and *limes* are believed to be of special value to people eating a high-fat/protein diet. These astringent fruits have antiseptic properties useful in controlling gut infections.

Oranges and *tangerines* share many of their healing properties, and both are good tonics for people suffering from poor appetite and sluggish digestion.

Warning: lemons and limes are highly acidic and are best avoided by people suffering from gastric ulcers.

COFFEE

Coffee has a mild laxative effect, but beware! Coffee contains caffeine, which can cause problems (*see page 28*).

CORIANDER SEEDS

Known for their healing qualities, these seeds stimulate digestion and are useful in the treatment of diarrhoea. Their ability to calm the bowel is thought helpful in the treatment of IBS.

CRANBERRIES

Known to contain antibacterial compounds that help control bladder infections, cranberries also help rid the gut of potentially harmful bacteria.

CUMIN

Add this flavourful spice to your cooking to control heartburn and wind.

DANDELION GREENS

The leaves of this unpopular weed are a healthy addition to a green salad because they contain substances thought to increase bile production and help detoxify the liver.

Always gather leaves from areas known to be free of herbicides, insecticides and other garden chemicals.

DATES

Well known as a gentle laxative helpful in preventing or treating constipation, dates are a good source of calcium, iron and potassium needed for healing.

The high sugar content in dates makes them an ideal ingredient in desserts and sweet meat dishes.

DILL

This is another ancient and effective aid to digestion. A few sprigs in a salad, or served on fish or poultry dishes, can reduce belching and flatulence and stimulate healthy digestion. Crushed dill seeds are a flavourful ingredient in salads, fish and meat dishes.

Some recipes for gripe water to treat babies with colic include an infusion of dill.

Remember: dill is a powerful herb and should be used in small amounts.

DRIED FRUIT (GENERAL)

Dried fruits are a good source of energy, nutrients and fibre needed to maintain a healthy gut. Used in moderation, they help prevent or treat constipation. By varying the amount eaten, colitis sufferers may find them a useful means of stabilizing their bowel.

Do not suddenly increase the amount of dried fruit in your diet. Begin eating dried fruit in small amounts and increasing as needed. Your bowel will tell you when you have found the ideal amount for you.

FENNEL

This much under-rated vegetable has a wonderful flavour and is well regarded for its healing powers by traditional Chinese and Ayurvedic practitioners. Known as an aid in the treatment of heartburn, wind, nausea and vomiting, fennel greatly benefits the digestive system.

All parts of the plant are used in cooking. The fleshy bulb and fine fern-like leaves can be incorporated into salads or cooked with fish and poultry. The bulb is delicious cooked and served as a side dish.

Fennel seeds are the plant's richest source of compounds that help control bloating and flatulence, and are frequently included as spices in Indian cooking. Chewed after dinner, they freshen the breath.

Adding fennel seeds to dishes made with cabbage helps control the flatulence sometimes caused by this important vegetable.

FIGS

Both fresh and dried figs contain ficin, thought to help digestion by calming the muscular activity of the gut. Their gentle laxative effect helps prevent chronic constipation. Nutritional therapists claim that figs benefit the stomach, pancreas and large intestine.

FISH

To maintain a healthy digestive system, enjoy oily fish rich in omega-3 fatty acids (mackerel, tuna, trout, herring, salmon and albacore) at least twice a week. Research evidence demonstrates the value of these essential fats in healing processes, and to the general well-being of the human body.

GARLIC (SEE ALSO 'ALLIUM')

An important item in nature's medicine cabinet, garlic has natural anti-viral and antibacterial properties that help control gastric infection. It has also been shown to help control blood cholesterol levels.

GINGER

Slices of preserved ginger, and foods containing reasonable quantities of fresh or ground ginger root, help control nausea associated with gastroenteritis, travel sickness, pregnancy and chemotherapy. Ginger also helps relieve heartburn, settle digestion, reduce wind and eliminate the feeling of bloating. Its benefits in the treatment of Crohn's disease, IBS and colitis have been reported. This peppery root helps prevent bad breath by cleaning the sinuses.

GRAPES

There are good reasons for giving grapes to people who are ill or infirm. Rich in easily digested sugars, they also contain useful amounts of substances believed to aid the immune system. In traditional Chinese medicine, grapes are thought to cleanse the liver, and are used as a remedy in cases of jaundice and hepatitis.

Phenols in grapes are thought to help combat the build-up of cholesterol in the blood. Red grapes are more potent than white (*see 'Berries and Red Grapes', page 38*).

HONEY

The healing nature of this food has been valued since biblical times. Recent scientific research suggests Manuka honey contains substances that inhibit the growth of *Helicobacter pylori*, the bacteria connected with gastric ulcers.

Ayurveda claims heating destroys honey's healing properties, making raw honey more valuable than commercial, blended products.

HORSERADISH

Able to stimulate the digestive processes, this ancient cooking ingredient makes an excellent accompaniment to meat, especially when combined in a sauce using live yoghurt.

Horseradish helps clear blocked sinuses, thus reducing the chance of developing bad breath.

KALE

Rich in fibre, vitamin C and B-vitamins, this unpopular vegetable is an excellent source of the sulphur compounds thought to heal gastric ulcers and help prevent bowel cancer.

KIWI FRUIT

Kiwi fruit contains soluble fibre needed to prevent constipation. The vitamin C and potassium, both well supplied by this fruit, support a healthy gut.

LENTILS

An excellent source of essential minerals, these pulses are packed with soluble fibre that helps prevent or relieve constipation. Some nutritional therapists suggest that lentils be included in the diet of those with coeliac disease.

LIVER

The healing effects of liver are considerable. Mouth ulcers and colitis have been shown to benefit from adding liver to the diet. Including this food in your diet at least once a week will support the general health of your own liver.

Sadly, liver has lost popularity over the years. Rich in vitamin A, most of the B-vitamins (including B12), vitamin D, copper, iron, molybdenum, selenium and zinc, liver supplies many of the nutrients essential for healthy digestive function. Calf, beef, lamb, chicken and pork liver are of equal value. Buy organic liver when possible, or limit yourself to liver from young animals when it is not. The liver is the body organ responsible for destroying toxic substances and storing those it cannot eliminate. The older an animal, the more likely it is to have built up a store of substances unsuitable for your own good health.

Remember: the high level of vitamin A in liver may be harmful to unborn children. Women who plan to get pregnant, or who are pregnant, should avoid liver until after delivery.

If you are taking vitamin A as a dietary supplement, liver should be eaten occasionally.

MELONS

A good source of vitamin C and betacarotene, melons are also a very useful source of pure fluid needed to maintain normal digestive functions.

MILLET

High in fibre, minerals and B-vitamins, millet is gluten free and a good food choice for people suffering from constipation and sensitivity to gluten (*see Crohn's disease, page 63*).

MINT (ALSO PEPPERMINT)

A favourite herb with many variations, all forms of mint help control bad breath and settle the digestive system. This may explain why sweets strongly flavoured with mint have been popular after-dinner treats for centuries. Used as ingredients in food, mint and mint oil have been shown to benefit cases of flatulence, Crohn's disease and IBS.

Leaf infusions, in the form of mint 'tea', help control an unsettled stomach (*see the recipe on page 221*).

NUTS (ALMONDS, BRAZIL NUTS, PINE KERNELS, WALNUTS AND EDIBLE SEEDS)

These foods are rich in B-vitamins, vitamin E, various minerals, oils and fibre needed for good gut health. Mouth ulcers may signal a borderline deficiency in B-vitamins, which can be corrected by adding nuts and seeds to the diet.

Brazil nuts are an excellent source of selenium, a mineral essential for good health. Research shows selenium levels are low in the British diet.

Remember: choking on nuts is as great a danger to young children as nut allergies.

NUTMEG

A spice popular across the globe, nutmeg helps control the discomfort of nausea. Add to sweets made with ginger and honey. Delicious when grated over cooked spinach.

OATS AND OAT BRAN

An excellent source of soluble fibre that helps prevent constipation and diverticulitis, oats have been shown to help control blood cholesterol levels. Oats are greatly valued in traditional medicine, and are used to heal abdominal bloating and indigestion, and to strengthen the pancreas.

Although gluten-free, oats do contain a substance that may cause bowel problems.

OLIVES AND EXTRA VIRGIN OLIVE OIL

Highly nutritious, olives are thought to contain natural healing substances that stimulate the release of bile from the gall bladder, lowering the risk of gallstones and improving liver function. Extra virgin oil contains higher levels of healing compounds than other grades of olive oil because it is from the first pressing of the fruit. Partnered with lemon juice in a dressing for green salads, fish or vegetables, olive oil aids digestion.

ONIONS (SEE 'ALLIUM')

OREGANO

This popular herb contains rosmarinic acid, a powerful anti-viral, antibacterial and anti-inflammatory compound that aids the digestive system.

PARSLEY

Enjoy eating the parsley garnish on your plate – it may be one of the most nutritious parts of the meal. A good source of nutrients including iron and vitamin C, parsley is rich in chlorophyll, a natural deodorant. Parsley helps prevent mouth odours when included in dishes containing members of the allium family. (Garlic butter is almost always made with lots of chopped parsley.) Parsley may help relieve colitis and is an aid to digestion.

Used for centuries as a natural diuretic, parsley aids the elimination of uric acid from the body.

PEARS

Pears should be a regular part of a healthy diet. They are a popular choice on many exclusion diets because they rarely cause allergies and are easy to digest. High in fibre and potassium, they are ideal food for preventing and treating constipation, and for people convalescing from illness.

Some nutritional therapists suggest pears are useful in the treatment of gall bladder disease.

PINEAPPLE

Rich in bromelain, known to help the breakdown and digestion of proteins, this fruit is thought to contain substances credited with blocking the formation of cancer-causing compounds (called nitrosamines) in the stomach.

Warning: pineapple should be avoided by people with gastric ulcers.

RASPBERRIES

Useful in the treatment of indigestion, liver conditions and diarrhoea, raspberries are rich in healing antibacterial compounds. An infusion made from raspberry leaves is often used to soothe the digestive system (*see 'Berries and Red Grapes', page 38*).

RICE

An excellent gluten-free food that helps control diarrhoea, rice is known to soothe the entire intestinal tract. A major source of easy-to-digest carbohydrate in the BRAT diet (*see page 26*), rice is an ideal food for people with coeliac disease. It is also thought to help people suffering from gallstones.

Brown rice is packed with essential B-vitamins, and its fibre helps relieve constipation. However, the tough outer husk may cause gut irritation and should be avoided by those known to have inflammation of the bowel.

ROSEMARY

Soothing to the digestive system in general, rosemary is used to relieve flatulence and indigestion.

RYE

Unless you are sensitive to gluten, rye is a good source of minerals and vitamins needed for a healthy gut, and makes a welcome change from bread and other baked products made with wheat. Rye is often used as a general aid to the pancreas, liver and gall bladder.

SAFFRON

Used in eastern cultures to help ease chronic diarrhoea, saffron is thought to be a rich source of natural antibacterial substances.

SAGE

Known to calm indigestion, sage is a good herb to use in dishes containing rich, heavy foods.

SAUERKRAUT

Having the same healing benefits as cabbage (*see page 40*), this pungent food also contains bacteria that may help digestion and maintain a healthy gut capable of extracting nutrients from food. (Sauerkraut is not a good choice for those on a low-sodium diet.)

STAR ANISE

Added to food, this exotic oriental spice helps control flatulence.

TARRAGON

A herb commonly used to help control belching, flatulence and stomach acidity.

TEA (BLACK, GREEN, OOLONG AND PEKOE)

A cup of tea helps fight infections. According to a research team at the Brigham and Women's Hospital in Boston, Massachusetts, these teas contain the amino acid

L-theanine, which appears to boost the activity of T-cells, the body's first line of defence against infection. People drinking 20 fluid ounces of tea per day (five to six cups) appeared to have stronger immune systems. Research by scientists in the United Kingdom suggests that five to six cups of green tea a day helps reduce blood pressure and lower cholesterol levels.

THYME

A popular herb, thyme helps control flatulence.

TOAST

White toast is a good source of easy-to-digest carbohydrate. Toast is part of the BRAT diet (*see page 26*) because it contains little fibre and is, therefore, a good food choice for those suffering from inflammatory bowel conditions or diarrhoea.

TURMERIC

Used for centuries as a liver tonic and treatment for ailments of the digestive system (ulcerative colitis, for example), turmeric contains curcumin, which gives the spice its brilliant yellow colour. Scientific evidence now suggests that this powerful substance acts as an antioxidant, an antimicrobial and an anti-inflammatory in the body.

WATERCRESS

Thought to be rich in natural antibiotics, watercress is used to relieve stomach upsets and colitis. People suffering side-effects from chemotherapy will profit from the high nutritional value of this tasty green plant.

Remember: wash watercress well, particularly before eating it raw.

WHEAT AND OTHER GRAINS (GENERAL)

Packed with fibre and carbohydrate energy, whole grains are an excellent source of B-vitamins, minerals, protein and unsaturated oils needed for a healthy gut. Most of these nutrients are located in the germ of the grain. (The germ is the fertile part of the grain that sends up a sprout when growth begins; most of the remainder of the seed is starch or outer husk.)

Products made with whole grain are coarse and heavy, and unattractive to many shoppers. To produce more pleasing, refined products, grains used to make flour are put through a 'milling' process that strips off the coarse outer husk of the kernel (bran). Unfortunately, the mineral- and vitamin-rich germ is lost in this process. A light sprinkling of wheat germ on cereals, soups, salads and baked goods can greatly increase your nutrient intake.

According the leading American nutritional therapist, Paul Pitchford, wheat absorbs a wider range of nutrients from the soil than other grains, and the balance of minerals in whole grain is similar to that of the human body. Therefore, of all the grains, whole-grain wheat makes an excellent part of a healthy diet.

In a small portion of the population, the gluten in wheat causes a severe medical condition known as coeliac disease (*see page 58*). Although controversy exists over the extent to which wheat also causes food intolerance and sensitivity, the best evidence suggests that this grain is a highly valuable food for the vast majority of people, young and old.

Remember: wheat, rye and barley contain gluten and should be avoided by people with coeliac disease and those who suffer from wheat intolerance.

YAMS AND SWEET POTATOES

Deliciously sweet and rich in fibre, these colourful root vegetables make a useful addition to your diet. Eating them once or twice a week will help you avoid constipation. They are thought to strengthen the pancreas and aid the body's sugar balance. Enjoy them in moderate-sized servings, because overindulging can lead to indigestion and bloating.

YOGHURT

Including bio yoghurt (live yoghurt) in your diet helps maintain a balance of healthy gut flora needed for digestion. It also discourages the growth of harmful yeasts, such as

Candida albicans. Live yoghurt helps restore the digestive system following a course of antibiotics, radiotherapy, chemotherapy or any other medical treatment that may disrupt the normal balance of gut bacteria (*see 'Probiotics', page 23*).

Healthy gut foods

Alliums – rich in antibacterial compounds
Chives
Garlic
Green onions
Onions
Shallots

Berries, red fruits and grapes– rich in natural antibacterial compounds
Bilberries
Blackcurrants
Blueberries
Cherries
Cranberries
Grapes
Raspberries

Citrus fruit – rich in vitamin C; stimulate digestion
Grapefruit
Lemons
Limes
Oranges

Fruits (other than berries and citrus fruit) – contain natural fibre, simple sugars, vitamins and minerals
Apples
Apricots

Avocados
Bananas
Dates
Figs
Grapes (red skinned)
Kiwi fruit
Melons
Pears
Pineapple

Green and leafy vegetables – for fibre, vitamins, minerals and healing compounds
Broccoli
Cabbage (and sauerkraut)
Celery
Chicory
Dandelion greens
Kale
Watercress

Herbs – for healing compounds that aid digestion
Basil
Camomile
Chervil
Dill
Fennel
Horseradish
Mint

Popular because of its high calcium and phosphorus content, yoghurt also contains riboflavin (vitamin B2) and vitamin B12 found in few other non-meat foods.

Oregano
Parsley
Rosemary
Sage
Tarragon
Thyme

Nuts and seeds – to add minerals, vitamins and essential fats to the diet
Almonds (almond oil)
Pine kernels
Sesame seeds
Walnuts

Olives and olive oil – to aid the liver and digestion

Pulses – for fibre
Lentils

Root vegetables – for fibre and healing plant compounds
Beetroot
Carrots
Sweet potatoes
Yams

Spices – contain compounds that aid digestion
Allspice
Black pepper
Caraway
Cardamom

Chilli
Cinnamon
Cumin
Fennel seeds
Ginger
Nutmeg
Saffron
Turmeric

Whole grains – for bulk, vitamins and minerals
Barley
Buckwheat
Millet
Oats
Rice
Rye
Wheat

Yoghurt – a natural probiotic

Other
Artichokes – an aid to the liver
Cheddar cheese
Honey
Liver
Oily fish – an excellent source of essential fatty acids
Tea (black, green, oolong and pekoe) – supports good gut health
Toast

five when things go wrong

It is a rare person who goes through life without experiencing the discomfort of mouth ulcers, heartburn, flatulence, nausea, diarrhoea and constipation. Usually these problems are of short duration and can be treated at home with sensible eating, rest and common sense. Unfortunately, more severe problems do occur, and about one in ten of us will suffer from a serious illness of the gut during some part of our lifetime. Symptoms and treatments vary, *but no matter what the complaint or illness, when things go wrong with the gut, food is part of the answer.*

Sometimes distinguishing between simple complaints and major illness of the gut can be difficult. A miserable bout of vomiting or heartburn can be self-limiting and cause only temporary distress, or these same conditions may be symptoms of more serious underlying diseases, such as food poisoning or a gastric ulcer. Similarly, feelings of bloating, nausea and bouts of diarrhoea are common complaints, but if these problems persist or reoccur over a period of time they could be signs of irritable bowel syndrome or Crohn's disease.

This chapter is divided into 20 sections. Each provides basic information about an illness of the digestive system and includes a brief description of symptoms, a list of useful healing foods, a list of foods to be avoided, and some facts about the illness. To help you include more healing foods in your diet, Marguerite Patten's healthy-gut recipes are recommended throughout.

If you suffer from a gut disorder and are under a doctor's care, check before changing your diet.

what is making you ill?

Maintaining a healthy gut obviously depends on eating the right food, but it is also essential to identify what makes you ill. Preventing a problem recurring takes some detective work. A bout of indigestion may have resulted from eating too quickly during a high-pressure lunch meeting with your boss. Or, if you live on a somewhat bland meat and potato diet, and go on holiday to a place where both the sun and food are hot, it would come as no surprise if your digestive system rebelled.

Creating an informal diary of your complaint is a good approach to identifying its cause. When a problem arises (halitosis, vomiting, heartburn, etc.) start your diary by writing down the relevant date, the time and the severity of the condition. Next, write down what you ate over the previous two meals, then briefly make a note of any event that may have triggered your distress. If the cause of your problem is not immediately obvious, keep the diary and add more information when symptoms return. Review your notes from time to time to see if you can identify a pattern. (Halitosis, or bad breath, may be a sign of a sinus or lung infection.)

You may be surprised by what you find. A smell in a particular place can trigger nausea (fish shops and counters are known to affect some people). Or your diary may show that recurring bouts of diarrhoea correspond with periods of unusual exertion during exercise (*see 'Athlete's Diarrhoea', page 66*). As much as you love crabmeat sandwiches, could they be contributing to your stomach cramps (*see page 31 for information about food intolerance*)? If a specific food seems to be the root of your problem, try an exclusion diet (*see page 31*).

Above all else, as you create your diary ask yourself one crucial question: Has anything in my life changed? Spotting a lifestyle change at the root of your new gastric distress can quickly point you in the direction of a prompt cure. Consider all aspects of your life. Are you smoking too much? Have your drinking habits changed? Are the children having problems at school? Are you feeling stressed because you suddenly find yourself caring for an ailing family member? Are you moving house, changing jobs, contemplating a divorce, or is there a new lover in your life?

Ask yourself about other aspects of your health. Has there been a change in your medication or method of birth control? Medication can affect the gut and cause uncomfortable – and sometimes serious – problems. Appendix Two provides basic information that can help you think about the pills you take and whether or not they may be having side-effects on your digestive system.

WARNING!

Seek help from your doctor at once if:
- you show signs of an acute allergic reaction (see *pages 30–1*).
- symptoms persist for more than a few days
- you develop a fever
- you experience intense abdominal pain
- there are signs of blood in vomit or stool (see *Glossary – 'false bleeding'*).

coeliac disease (malabsorption syndrome, sprue)

Coeliac disease reduces the effectiveness of the small intestine, and curtails the normal transfer of nutrients from the gut to the body. Approximately 1 in 300 Europeans suffer from this debilitating condition. It is caused by an intolerance to gluten, a natural protein occurring in wheat, rye and barley, and the incidence of the disease seems to increase with the expanded use of these cereals in processed foods. Although debated, some experts suspect that oats contain a substance similar to gluten, and advise coeliac sufferers to avoid oats as well. There is no cure, but a healthy diet free from all traces of gluten helps rebuild and sustain a healthier gut.

HEALING FOODS

- *Rice, polenta (cornmeal), wild rice, millet, quinoa, buckwheat, amaranth*
- *Potatoes*
- *Fresh fruit*
- *Vegetables*
- *Dairy foods and eggs*

- *Meat, fish, poultry and cheese made without fillers or sauces containing gluten*
- *Arrowroot or flour made from rice, corn or potatoes for thickening*
- *Speciality foods trusted to be 'gluten-free'*

FOODS TO AVOID

All foods containing wheat, rye and barley, including pasta, cereal, couscous, semolina, barley water, fondants, canned soups and other products thickened with wheat flour. Unless specifically labelled as gluten-free, processed cheeses, stock cubes, gravy granules, mustards and other cooking products are all likely to contain gluten. Unlike 20 years ago, gluten-free alternatives are now widely available and the majority are very good and getting better all the time. If you tried gluten-free products a few years ago and were disappointed, try again.

Remember: oats may affect some coeliac patients.

USEFUL RECIPES

Roast Fish with Herb Sauce (page 118)
Rice Pudding (page 194)

DID YOU KNOW?

- *Symptoms of coeliac disease include bloating, indigestion, weakness, weight loss and anaemia due to progressive malnutrition. Stools are usually large and may contain fat. Glossitis – an inflammation of that part of the throat associated with the voice box – may also occur.*
- *Coeliac disease leads to malabsorption syndrome. Malabsorption occurs when the tiny villi in the intestine are damaged, reduced in size or flattened. As the villi are responsible for absorbing and transporting nutrients from within the gut, their inability to function denies the body much-needed proteins, vitamins and minerals. (*For more information about malabsorption, see page 13.*)*
- *The disease develops in all age groups, but is most common in infants and during the third, fifth and sixth decades. If weaned early, infants can develop coeliac disease soon after they are introduced to cereals. This inability to cope with gluten may have few symptoms or may cause considerable upset. As an affected infant grows, the digestive system matures and digesting cereals is soon no longer a concern. There is some evidence that a genetic factor may determine*

which children experience this problem. This factor would remain for life. It is possible that adults who develop coeliac disease may have carried this genetic weakness into old age, when the body's functions slow. If this slow-down involves the digestive mechanisms that allow us to cope with gluten, the risk of coeliac disease increases.

colitis

Colitis is an inflammation of the colon and rectum causing pain, bloating, diarrhoea and, in severe cases, bleeding. The condition may be acute or chronic, and in severe cases causes ulceration of the lining of the lower gut (*see 'Ulcerative Colitis', page 82*). Most sufferers may have few symptoms, while others may be prostrate from the illness and require surgery. Altering the diet can significantly improve symptoms.

HEALING FOODS

- *Foods high in soluble fibre* (see page 21)
- *Apples and other fruit*
- *Berries*
- *Parsley*
- *Watercress and other green leafy vegetables*
- *Oily fish*
- *Liver*
- *Low-fat dairy products*
- *Yoghurt (live)*
- *Foods rich in zinc, such as eggs, Cheddar cheese and beef steak*
- *Foods high in nutritional value*

FOODS TO AVOID

- *All foods high in insoluble fibre* (see page 21)
- *Foods to which you know you have an intolerance*
- *All forms of bran*
- *Nuts and seeds*
- *Sweetcorn*
- *Junk food*

USEFUL RECIPES

Liver Pâté (page 95)
Oeufs à la Tripe (page 172)

DID YOU KNOW?

- *Colitis reduces the body's ability to absorb nutrients from the gut, so choose foods high in nutritional value such as liver, dark green leafy vegetables and dried fruit, which will provide protein, vitamins A, C, D and B12, and minerals including iron, zinc and calcium. (For more about nutrients, see page 29.)*
- *Increasing evidence suggests that colitis results from inflammation caused by an immune response, possibly to certain foods.*
- *This illness was thought to be psychosomatic in origin, but recent evidence points to a physiological cause.*
- *Colitis affects about 4–6 people in 100,000; onset is usually between the mid-20s and mid-life.*

constipation

Constipation is not an illness, but a common sign that the large bowel is having trouble getting rid of waste. It is normal to have one or two bowel motions a day. The normal stool (product of a bowel motion) is large, formed and soft and causes neither straining nor discomfort. Constipation is characterized by passing fewer stools, which are hard and dry (described as 'rabbit droppings' or 'bullets') and frequently accompanied by straining and discomfort.

Constipation may be a symptom of a more serious condition, such as irritable bowel syndrome.

HEALING FOODS

- *Increase your fluid intake. You should drink between seven and eight glasses (2 litres/3½ pints) of water a day. This should be increased if you are losing large amounts of fluid through perspiration or participate in strenuous activities.*

- *For simple constipation, gradually increase your intake of foods high in fibre, especially whole-grain products, green leafy vegetables, fresh fruit, dried apricots, figs, dates and prunes. Eating yams, parsnips or sweet potatoes once or twice a week can work wonders. All these foods have a high nutritional content. Bran can be added to the diet for bulk, but contains few nutrients and can cause flatulence and discomfort when used in large quantities.*
- *When constipation is a symptom of a more serious illness, see the advice given under that heading. In general, if the problem is serious, increase the amount of soluble fibre in your diet (see page 21), and avoid harsh, insoluble fibre like that found in bran, whole grains, nuts and seeds.*
- *Remember that tea, coffee and cola drinks act as mild diuretics. They should not be included when you estimate your daily fluid intake because they stimulate fluid loss, rather than restore it.*

FOODS TO AVOID

A low-fibre diet is the most common cause of constipation. Avoid a diet dominated by dairy products, meat and highly refined carbohydrates, such as cake and baked goods made with highly processed white flour.

USEFUL RECIPES

Lime and Mint Lentil Loaf (page 143)
Hummus (page 97)
Vegetable and Nut Risotto (page 169)
Flapjacks (page 214)

DID YOU KNOW?

- *Experts claim constipation is so common in Western society that it is taken almost for granted. People living on diets based largely on fruits and vegetables, like those in Asia and Africa, are rarely affected. It is also true that they rarely suffer from conditions of the colon now commonly experienced by many eating low-fibre/high-fat foods.*
- *The elderly and pregnant women tend to suffer more from constipation than others. Gradually increasing the amount of high-fibre foods will resolve the problem.*
- *Putting off going to the toilet is a common cause of constipation. Avoiding using public toilets while on holiday or out shopping can lead to problems. If you are worried about hygiene, carry toilet seat covers and antibacterial wipes with you.*

- *Iron tablets can cause constipation. If you think this may be your problem, try increasing the fibre in your diet. If that does not work, ask your chemist to suggest a gentle laxative. Do not stop taking prescribed iron tablets without advice from your doctor.*
- *Common causes of constipation include: lack of exercise, depression, an underactive thyroid, and certain medications such as diuretics, morphine, codeine, and some antidepressants. Some pain medication contains codeine (Co-codamol and Co-dydramol are examples) and can cause constipation.*
- *Constipation is no joke. It can set the scene for far more serious conditions such as haemorrhoids and anal fissures (small tears) leading to pain and bleeding when having a bowel motion. Prolonged cases can result in faecal impaction and rectal prolapse. Experts think constipation may contribute to diverticular disease (see page 67).*
- *Contrary to many statements in the lay press, constipation does not cause the release of toxins responsible for nausea, furred tongue, fatigue and depression. According to the Royal Society of Medicine Health Encyclopaedia, these symptoms result from an awareness of a full rectum and a belief that constipation is harmful.*

crohn's disease (regional ileitis)

Crohn's disease is an inflammatory disease that can attack any part of the gastrointestinal system, from the mouth to lower bowel. In the intestine it attacks both the superficial and inner layers of the intestinal wall. Common symptoms include nausea, pain, fever, chills, diarrhoea and weakness. It may be caused by an immune reaction.

HEALING FOODS

- *Live yoghurt (see 'Probiotics', page 23)*
- *Both ginger and mint tea may be soothing (see recipes on page 221)*

FOODS TO AVOID

- *Keep a food diary and see if you can spot foods that 'trigger' symptoms. Many experts advise that all dairy products, meat, eggs, tea, coffee and alcohol should be totally eliminated from the diet. (Lactose intolerance is a common problem; see page 31.)*
- *During a flare-up, reduce the fibre in your diet.*

- *Reduce refined sugar in your diet.*
- *Oily fish, rich in omega-3 fatty acids, are good for the gut, but may be a negative factor in some Crohn's disease cases.*

USEFUL RECIPES

Fruit Smoothies made with live yoghurt and berries (page 218)
Courgette and Mint Soup (page 106)
Buckwheat and Fruit Salsa (page 149)

DID YOU KNOW?

- *Bacteria may play a role in this disease, so cook food well.*
- *Crohn's disease frequently begins during adolescence.*
- *The cause of this illness remains a mystery, but many experts believe the condition involves an autoimmune response within the gut, possibly precipitated by a food intolerance.*
- *Although Crohn's disease usually begins in the gut, complications can occur including arthritis, gallstones, kidney stones, skin swellings, and fusion of the bones of the spinal column (ankylosing spondylitis).*

diarrhoea

Diarrhoea is not an illness, but a symptom that the gut is not working properly. It is characterized by the passage of watery, loose stools, usually caused by the failure of the large intestine to absorb adequate water from the stool. This failure may result from the effects of infection (food poisoning, dysentery, typhoid, for example), toxins and poisons, medications (including strong or excessive use of laxatives) and underlying conditions, such as irritable bowel syndrome.

HEALING FOODS

- *Diarrhoea can cause dehydration, and may have serious consequences for both the young and the elderly. Rehydration products are available at most chemists, but if you need to make your own, see the section on vomiting, below.*
- *If you have a prolonged bout of diarrhoea, or feel especially unwell, you may not feel like*

eating. However, consuming small quantities of mashed banana will help restore your mineral balance and provide the carbohydrate energy you need. After a few hours, take good advice from scientists at Harvard University and stay on the BRAT diet for 24–48 hours (see pages 26–7).

- *Camomile tea and foods containing peppermint can help ease the cramps that sometimes accompany diarrhoea.*

FOODS TO AVOID

- *Foods that may be contaminated or contain dangerous bacteria.*
- *Excess caffeine – this can cause diarrhoea in some people.*
- *Too many high-fibre foods – these can cause loose motions; 30 grams of fibre a day should be adequate.*

USEFUL RECIPES

Toast, plain or topped with banana, ginger syrup or other appetizing spread (page 181)
Mint tea (page 221)
Chicken and Almond Soup (page 107)
Summer Berry Smoothie (page 219)

DID YOU KNOW?

- *Diarrhoea is a common complaint that may indicate a more complex problem.*
- *Many people are reluctant to discuss diarrhoea, and so suffer without appropriate care. Remember that diarrhoea can lead to the loss of fluids and the nutrients potassium and sodium, resulting in weakness – and even mental confusion – associated with abnormal blood chemistry. Anaemia, weight loss and dehydration can also occur.*
- *Sometimes the stool is very soft but not watery – this is known as a 'loose motion'. Loose motions can be caused by eating an unusual amount of fatty or oily foods, or by eating too many high-fibre foods or foods to which you have a mild intolerance, such as cow's milk and dairy products. These may be embarrassing and uncomfortable, but diarrhoea is more serious.*
- *Diarrhoea can be acute, lasting one or two days. It can also be chronic and go on for weeks. Chronic diarrhoea can result from a long-standing disease, an infection of the gut by a parasite or fungus, or be a side-effect of medication. If you are on a prescribed drug – especially an antibiotic – for an extended period of time and begin suffering diarrhoea, read*

the information sheet that came with your medication, or ask your chemist for advice about whether your prescription may be causing the problem (see pages 226–30 for more information about how medication can affect the gut). *Food poisoning is a common cause of diarrhoea (see 'Vomiting' and pages 73 and 222–5 for more information). A major dietary change, excessive amounts of fatty foods, medications, and both physical and mental stress can all increase the risk of this distressing condition.*

- *Travellers often suffer from stomach upset when they make rapid dietary changes or encounter foods that may introduce new strains of bacteria into their gut. Given a few days in one place, digestive problems cease when the body adapts to these new conditions.*

- *A gluten-free or dairy-free diet can be the answer for some people suffering chronic diarrhoea (see pages 30–31 for more information).*

- *The overuse of laxatives can cause harmful diarrhoea. Never use laxatives for any purpose other than help with stubborn constipation; never use laxatives as part of a slimming programme.*

- *Chronic diarrhoea is a symptom of several serious gut conditions, including Crohn's disease, coeliac disease and irritable bowel syndrome. Read more about these illnesses under the appropriate heading.*

- *Chronic or blood-streaked diarrhoea should be reported to your GP at once.*

athlete's diarrhoea

Runners and other athletes often find they suffer from a sudden rush from the bowels. During exercise, blood is diverted from the gut to muscle tissue, thus slowing the absorption of nutrients from the intestine. As a consequence, these nutrients then draw water from the body into the gut, causing diarrhoea. Suffering from Crohn's disease, ulcerative colitis or food intolerances can make matters worse.

Drink water before strenuous exercise, but do so in moderation. When preparing for a race or extended run, cut down on high-fibre foods, fatty foods, dried fruit, caffeine and foods containing high levels of vitamin C.

If you suffer from athlete's diarrhoea to the point where it interferes with your sport, seek advice from a professional trained in sports medicine.

diverticulitis

When pressure builds up within the lower bowel (colon) and expands its width, as happens during constipation, weakened areas of the muscular walls may bulge out into pockets or pouches: these are called diverticula. Inflammation and/or infection in these areas are called diverticulitis. Low-fibre diets are thought to be the main cause of this potentially dangerous condition.

HEALING FOODS

- *See the section on Constipation (page 61)*
- *Drink plenty of water!*
- *Apples*
- *Berries – these are high in natural antibacterial substances*
- *Cooked green leafy vegetables*
- *Foods rich in soluble fibre, including oats and brown rice*
- *Camomile tea*
- *Live yoghurt*

FOODS TO AVOID

- *Forgo foods made with highly refined carbohydrates, specifically table sugar and white flour.*
- *Skip the fatty meals; it is best to leave the burgers and shakes or deep-fried cod and chips for the occasional meal, and not make them a regular part of your diet.*

USEFUL RECIPES

Oatmeal and Watercress Soup (page 112)
Baked Apples (page 199)
Pineapple and Apple Crisp (page 196)

DID YOU KNOW?

- *About half the population over 50 have diverticular pouches in their gut, but they are asymptomatic and cause no problems. Problems arise only when circumstances cause inflammation of tissue within the pouch.*

- *You can protect your lower bowel from developing chronic constipation by drinking plenty of water and eating foods high in soluble fibre, such as oat bran.*
- *Symptoms of acute diverticulitis are sharp pain in the lower left abdomen accompanied by fever and constipation.*
- *Experts link diverticulitis with the low-fibre Western diet. As more people around the world replace traditional diets, rich in fruits and vegetables, with high-fat foods based on refined carbohydrates, this illness is on the increase.*
- *Middle-aged people and the elderly are most susceptible to this condition. More women than men are sufferers.*

flatulence

The rumble of sometimes smelly gas released from the colon can be mortifying. Here are some tips on how you can avoid this embarrassment.

HEALING FOODS

- *Increase your intake of live yoghurt (see 'Probiotics', page 23).*
- *Drink herbal teas, such as peppermint and fennel.*
- *Add flavour to your cooking by using more caraway, cardamom, fennel and thyme. These seeds add flavour to many dishes – try crushed fennel seeds in warm potato salad, for example.*
- *Rice is easier to digest than other complex carbohydrates and produces very little gas. If flatulence is a major problem, try substituting rice and rice flour in your cooking.*

FOODS TO AVOID

Reduce your intake of cabbage, peas, lentils and beans. Remember that these foods are rich sources of fibre needed to help elimination from the bowel and avoid constipation (*see pages 61–2*). Make sure you replace any 'culprits' with other high-fibre foods, including wholegrain bread, fresh fruits and vegetables. Bran added to foods can also help but should be used with caution: too much may encourage other problems.

USEFUL RECIPES

Salmon Broth (page 113)
Moroccan Fish with Dates (page 116)
Fruit Soup – Apple variation (page 109)

DID YOU KNOW?

- *Passing air is a normal result of digestion; most of the time you are unaware it happens. The digestive processes in a normal adult produce more than 20 litres of gas per day; happily, most is consumed by bacteria in the lower gut, and only about 5 litres are expelled.*
- *The habit of swallowing air increases the amount of flatulence.*
- *Rapid eating and drinking increases air swallowing and the risk of excessive flatulence.*
- *Stress can increase air swallowing, and thus both belching and flatulence.*

gallstones

Gallstones are lumps of mineral salts, bile pigment or cholesterol that accumulate in the gall bladder (*see page 12*). They can be as small as a grain of sand or larger than a marble. Symptoms range from mild upper abdominal discomfort in the upper right-hand quadrant to severe pain with vomiting. Many people have gallstones without experiencing symptoms (silent stones).

HEALING FOODS

- *Oats, pasta, rice, wholegrain bread and other foods high in soluble fibre*
- *Fresh fruit and vegetables*
- *Artichokes*
- *Extra virgin olive oil*

FOODS TO AVOID

- *Fatty meat*
- *Full-fat dairy products*
- *Chocolates*

- *Rich sauces*
- *Ice cream and other fatty desserts*

USEFUL RECIPES

Waldorf Salad (page 99)
Aïöli (page 156)
Penne with Stir-fry Vegetables (page 165)

DID YOU KNOW?

- *Factors associated with gallstones include:*
  - *A diet high in refined carbohydrate*
  - *A diet high in saturated fats*
  - *High oestrogen levels*
  - *Cholesterol-reducing drugs*
  - *Obesity*
  - *Diabetes*
- *Vegetarians are less prone to gallstones than those who eat large quantities of red meat.*
- *Stones can pass naturally down the bile duct (a small tube extending from the gall bladder into the gut); this is called 'biliary colic' and can cause considerable pain.*
- *Stones sometimes block the flow of secretions from the pancreas into the gut, causing jaundice and occasionally a dangerous condition called pancreatitis.*
- *Three times more women are affected than men.*
- *Age matters. The elderly are those most likely to suffer from gallstones.*

gastric ulcers (peptic ulcers, duodenal ulcers)

(*See also 'Indigestion', page 75.*)

Ulcers develop in the upper digestive tract when the mucous lining becomes inflamed and breaks down. Peptic ulcers occur in the main body of the stomach. Ulcers found just beyond the stomach, in the small area where it joins the small intestine, are called duodenal ulcers. Recent medical research indicates that the bacterium *Helicobacter pylori* and the use of non-steroidal anti-inflammatory drugs (NSAIDs) play a large part in the formation of most ulcers.

HEALING FOODS

- *Apricots*
- *Blackcurrants*
- *Blueberries*
- *Strawberries*
- *Cabbage*
- *Green leafy vegetables*
- *Peppers, red and green (if your stomach allows)*
- *Cheddar cheese*
- *Wholegrain products*
- *Eggs*
- *Seafood, especially oily fish and oysters*
- *Live yoghurt* (see 'Probiotics', page 23)

FOODS TO AVOID

- *Salted and smoked foods*
- *Spicy and salty sauces – soya, Worcestershire, HP, etc.*
- *Pickles*
- *Caffeinated drinks – coffee, tea, cola*
- *Chilli peppers*
- *Black pepper*
- *Alcoholic beverages*
- *Foods high in refined sugar, fats or salt*

USEFUL RECIPES

Cheese Soup made with Cheddar cheese (page 105)
Spiced Coleslaw (page 140)
Yoghurt Lemon Syllabub – substitute berries for lemon (page 184)
Eggy Bread (page 174)

- *Pain in the centre part of the upper abdomen, just below the ribs, is the characteristic symptom of gastric ulcers. Pain increases with hunger. Nausea may occur.*
- *Smoking and alcohol are both risk factors for gastric ulcers.*
- Helicobacter pylori *is the bacterium found in the stomach of many ulcer patients. It causes inflammation that may lead to gastritis and ulcers. Eating more black and blue berries, and other foods known to contain natural antibacterial compounds, is thought to help fight this infection.*
- *Foods rich in betacarotene, vitamin C and zinc are thought to help heal gastric ulcers. (For more information about specific foods, see pages 35–55.)*
- *It may surprise you to learn that modern experts advocate eating smallish meals based on a normal diet; the old days of poached fish, milky bread and low-fibre meals are over.*
- *Studies suggest that oily fish, rich in the omega-3 fatty acids, aid healing (see page 45 for more information).*

gastritis

This is a common symptom caused by inflammation of the stomach lining. Sufferers experience a burning or 'grinding' sensation in the upper abdomen that may move into the chest. Gas and nausea sometimes accompany this pain.

HEALING FOODS

- *Drink plenty of water.*
- *Eat light foods with few spices for a day or two.*
- *Foods on the BRAT diet.*

FOODS TO AVOID

- *Acidic foods, including citrus fruit (orange juice) and pickles*
- *Milk*
- *Fatty food*
- *Alcohol*
- *Drinks containing caffeine and fizzy drinks*

Smoothies made with live yoghurt and fruit (page 218)
Toast with a topping of your choice (pages 180–2)
Chicken and Almond Soup (page 107)

DID YOU KNOW?

- *Risk factors include stress, overeating, too much caffeine, smoking, excess alcohol, bacterial or viral infections and certain medications.* (See pages 226–30 for more information about how medication can affect your gut.)
- *Milk protein can trigger gastritis in people suffering from lactose intolerance* (see page 31).

gastroenteritis

Gastroenteritis is an infection of the gut in which dangerous organisms destroy or crowd out the healthy bacteria needed for normal digestion. It is also known as food poisoning, and the primary symptoms are vomiting, diarrhoea and weakness due to fluid loss.

For basic advice on what to eat after an attack, read the preceding section on diarrhoea (*page 64*) and follow the BRAT diet for the first 48 hours after symptoms cease (*see page 26*). Subsequent to the BRAT diet, make sure you eat live yoghurt at least twice a day to help restore the balance of normal intestinal bacteria. Also enjoy dark berries and red grapes for their antibacterial benefits. Frozen packets of summer fruits are now available in most large supermarkets, and can be a handy source of natural healing even in the depths of winter.

'Smoothies' made with live yoghurt and berries are an easy-to-digest way to a healthier gut. If you do not already enjoy these delicious treats, Marguerite Patten has written some smoothie recipes to get you started.

USEFUL RECIPES

In addition to the suggestions above, try:

Fruit Soup – substitute berries for mango (page 108)

Accompany food with *Roast Garlic* (page 142) or *Onion Marmalade* (page 146), and take advantage of their natural antibacterial content.

halitosis (bad breath)

Foul-smelling breath can result from smoking, the consumption of alcohol, poor dental hygiene and eating strong-smelling foods such as garlic and onions. If none of these habits apply to you, and you have persistent bad breath, check with your doctor as the cause may be gum disease, tonsillitis, an abscessed tooth, or a lung or sinus infection.

HEALING FOODS

- *Mint and parsley both contain high levels of the natural deodorant chlorophyll. Eating the garnish of fresh parsley on your dinner plate will help keep your breath fresh and add to your intake of vitamins and minerals.*
- *Chewing raw vegetables helps maintain strong gums and teeth.*
- *If you suffer from a sinus condition, horseradish, mustard and ginger will help decongest the airways.*

FOODS TO AVOID

Garlic, onions, shallots and other alliums are packed with natural antibacterial compounds and are increasingly respected for their healing benefits. To counter their 'pong', eat parsley at the same meal.

USEFUL RECIPES

Parsley Sauce (page 152)
Waldorf Salad (page 99)

- *Bad breath can be the sign of a serious illness: a fishy or ammonia smell may indicate liver problems; the smell of acetone may indicate a serious diabetic condition.*
- *Some women experience 'menstrual breath' around the time of their period. Regular brushing of teeth, mint tea and eating raw foods with high chlorophyll content (parsley, watercress, spinach) can help eliminate the problem.*
- *Mouth ulcers may contribute to bad breath, especially during menstruation (see 'Mouth Ulcers', below).*
- *Although both constipation and indigestion are said to cause bad breath, the medical evidence for this is slim.*

heartburn/indigestion (gastro-oesophageal reflux)

Heartburn (indigestion) occurs when an excess of acid rises from the stomach into the oesophagus (gullet), causing burning pain. Occasionally, stomach acid reaches the mouth, leaving a repellent bitter taste. Symptoms include pain in the left side of the chest or below the breastbone, upper abdominal discomfort, bloating, nausea, belching and wind (flatulence).

HEALING FOODS

- *Mint in all forms, including soothing mint tea. Mint sauce (made with real mint leaves) eaten as part of a fatty meal may help prevent an attack of indigestion.*
- *Cook with cardamom, caraway, chervil, cumin, dill, fennel and ginger.*
- *A cup of camomile tea at bedtime helps soothe a delicate stomach.*

FOODS TO AVOID

- *If you drink alcohol, do so in moderation.*
- *Certain raw salad foods – onions, radishes, cucumbers.*
- *Acidic foods such as pickles, vinegar and lemon juice.*
- *Fatty foods – skip the fry-ups, milkshakes and the greasy burgers.*
- *Chilli peppers and hot, spicy foods.*
- *Some people find chocolate, tea and coffee make gastric acidity worse.*
- *Do not eat cheese before bedtime.*

USEFUL RECIPES

Lentil Soup (page 110)
Courgette and Mint Soup (page 106)
Mint Tea (page 221)

DID YOU KNOW?

- *Primary causes of indigestion are eating too much, eating the wrong foods, eating too fast and stress.*
- *Indigestion is one of the most common forms of gastrointestinal distress. It frequently occurs after meals, especially large fatty dinners (a plague during the holiday season).*
- *Lying down after eating makes matters worse. If you tend to have indigestion, and have just eaten a large meal, take a walk rather than a nap.*
- *Indigestion occurs in all age groups, including infants.*
- *Small meals eaten at regular intervals can help control this painful condition.*
- *If you smoke – stop. Nicotine stimulates the flow of acid gastric juices.*
- *The pain of heartburn can cause such acute chest pain it may be mistaken by the victim for a heart attack.*
- *Persistent indigestion and heartburn should be discussed with your doctor. Over a long period, repeated bouts of heartburn can cause erosion or ulceration of the oesophagus, leading to a narrowing of the gut and difficulty in swallowing.*
- *Pregnancy and obesity can contribute to heartburn by changing the normal placement of the stomach.*
- *Hiatus hernia (see below) may cause heartburn.*

hiatus hernia

A hiatus hernia develops when a part of the stomach pushes up from the abdomen into the chest cavity through a weakened part of the muscle forming the diaphragm. It can cause considerable pain that may mimic a heart attack.

HEALING FOODS

- *Enjoy more and smaller meals during the day. Keep foods light.*

FOODS TO AVOID

- *Heavy meals dominated by fatty and highly spiced ingredients.*

DID YOU KNOW?

Circumstances that encourage the formation of a hiatus hernia include:

- *obesity*
- *pregnancy*
- *tight belts and waistbands*

inflammatory bowel disease (IBD)

This is a general term used to describe both ulcerative colitis and Crohn's disease. More information about these diseases is provided under their separate headings.

Many people afflicted by these disorders are lactose intolerant and advised to avoid dairy products. However, special products on the market get around this problem. Lactase, the enzyme needed to digest dairy products, can be purchased as drops and in capsules, and milk treated with lactase is available.

irritable bowel syndrome (IBS, spastic colon)

This is one of the most difficult illnesses of the digestive system to manage because it produces pain and other symptoms without having a clinically identifiable organic cause. On examination, the bowel walls show no bleeding or inflammation, unlike inflammatory bowel disease (IBD), with which it is often confused (see above). IBS is widespread and can be very debilitating.

HEALING FOODS

- *Live yoghurt (read about probiotics on page 23)*
- *Fresh fruit*

- *Vegetables*
- *Globe artichokes*
- *Drink plenty of water (at least 3 litres/5 pints a day)*
- *Mint, camomile and lemon balm teas*
- *Ginger*
- *Coriander seeds ground and added to appropriate dishes*

FOODS TO AVOID

- *Any food to which you know you have an intolerance*
- *Wholegrain foods and pulses*
- *Bran*
- *Fatty foods, including cheese, butter, ice cream and red meat*
- *Foods known to cause flatulence – beans, lentils and cabbage, for example*
- *Coffee, tea and cola*
- *AVOID LARGE MEALS: eat small, frequent meals that do not 'overfill' your intestine*

USEFUL RECIPES

Fruit Soup made with Apples (page 109)

Yoghurt Dressing (page 162)

Tajine of Quail (page 136)

Cranachan (page 186)

DID YOU KNOW?

- *IBS is a common complaint and accounts for about half the cases of bowel conditions that lead to seeking medical help. It is estimated that one in three people in the UK suffers bouts of this illness from time to time.*
- *Symptoms vary and can include one or more of the following: flatulence, alternating diarrhoea and constipation, nausea, a sensation of bloating, feelings of urgency and an inability to empty the bowel. Bleeding can occur. If this happens, seek medical help at once.*
- *No organic cause has been identified, but an attack often occurs during a period of stress: business or marital problems, bereavement and money worries are examples.*
- *IBS affects three times more women than men, and usually begins between the ages of 20 and 40. Its symptoms include a feeling of bloating, pain (usually in one corner of the abdomen),*

alternating diarrhoea and constipation, flatulence, headache, and feelings of anxiety. Eating may bring on pain and urgency to empty the bowels. Both the small and large intestine may be involved. Medical investigations are typically negative, except that muscular activity in the colon is abnormally rapid.

- *Some medical experts continue to advise IBS patients to eat high-fibre diets, usually bulked up with bran. Recent scientific evidence has shown, however, that bran and high-fibre diets can make matters worse.*
- *If you have a food intolerance, adapt your diet accordingly. Keeping a food diary can help you identify which foods may trigger an attack.*
- *Include more live yoghurt in your diet; the healthy bacteria will help heal inflamed intestines.*
- *Foods that produce flatulence can irritate this condition* (see page 68 for more information).
- *Skip drinks that contain caffeine, and substitute herbal teas that soothe the nerves and stomach. Caffeine is a stimulant that heightens the effects of stress.*
- *Eat regular and small meals.*
- *IBS is diagnosed by excluding other illnesses. Make sure you seek medical help if symptoms are severe, and always seek medical advice in the case of rectal bleeding.*
- *Some IBS sufferers find aloe vera soothes inflammation and reduces symptoms. Many people find aloe vera has an unpleasant taste and prefer to take it in capsule form; however, the liquid supplement may have a higher potency. Read the product information and use your personal requirements to determine your choice.*

mouth ulcers (apthous ulcers)

Ulcers occurring inside the mouth are painful and can interfere with normal chewing. Affected areas appear white, grey or yellowish with raised red borders. They can occur anywhere in the mouth: gums, roof, floor, tongue, or inside the cheeks. If located in or near the entrance to the throat, ulcers can cause considerable pain that may mimic earache.

HEALING FOODS

- *Foods rich in B-vitamins (wheatgerm, whole grains, nuts)*
- *Foods rich in zinc (nuts, wheatgerm, eggs, shellfish)*
- *Foods rich in folic acid (dark-green vegetables, whole grains)*
- *If you are anaemic, foods rich in iron (apricots, fortified breakfast cereal, liver, dark chocolate)*

FOODS TO AVOID

Mouth ulcers are aggravated by acidic foods, such as vinegar and pickles, salty foods, alcohol and sucking boiled sweets.

USEFUL RECIPES

Liver with Prunes and Herbs (page 129)
Soufflé Omelette with Fruit (page 178)

DID YOU KNOW?

- *Common causes are nutritional deficiency, stress and food sensitivities, but mouth ulcers may also appear during an attack of Herpes simplex, Crohn's disease, ulcerative colitis and coeliac disease.*
- *If you bite your tongue or the inside of your mouth, rinse with a weak solution of antiseptic mouthwash; repeat every four hours until the soreness disappears.*
- *Check the state of your dental health: broken teeth can cut into the tender tissues lining the mouth.*
- *Grinding your teeth during sleep can also cause soft-tissue injury.*
- *High temperatures and immuno-suppressant drugs may cause mouth ulcers.*
- *Some women suffer from mouth ulcers around the time of their period; these may contribute to bad breath.*
- ***Warning***: *mouth ulcers can resemble the early stages of oral cancer. If you have an ulcer that persists for more than a month, see your doctor or dentist.*

nausea

Nausea, or feeling sick, is a common symptom associated with many illnesses and conditions including hormonal changes during the early months of pregnancy, food poisoning, excessive intake of food or drink, side-effects of certain medications, stress, travel motion and Crohn's disease. This unpleasant sensation usually precedes vomiting.

HEALING FOODS

- *Ginger: an ancient plant widely known for its healing properties, ginger is a great aid in controlling nausea. Nibbling a piece of candied ginger, or eating one or two sweet biscuits flavoured with ginger nibs, are good ways to control travel sickness and the nausea that can accompany the first few months of pregnancy. Even the nausea caused by chemotherapy may be treated with this powerful spice.*
- *Fennel: a herb tasting of aniseed, the seeds and feathery leaves of which are used to aid digestion and control nausea. The taste of fennel marries well with fish. Small slices of fresh fennel add delicious crunch to a salad, or will cook well in a soup or stew.*
- *Nutmeg: used in small quantities, this powerful spice helps control nausea. Try grating a small amount into a hot cup of ginger and honey tea.*
- *Camomile tea helps soothe nausea.*

FOODS TO AVOID

- *Any food you know triggers nausea.*
- *Tainted foods, or foods that may have been cooked or stored in less than hygienic conditions* (see pages 222–5 for information on food hygiene).

USEFUL RECIPES

Ginger Milk Shake (page 220)
Toast with Ginger Syrup (page 181)
Spiced Vegetable Salsa (page 150)
Ginger Carrot Cake (page 216)

DID YOU KNOW?

- *The word* nausea *has its roots in the Greek word* naus, *meaning a ship.*
- *When you suffer from nausea, eat small, frequent meals.*
- *Make sure you are drinking enough water, but sip it rather than gulping it down.*
- *If you know you feel ill because you ate or drank too much, the answer is obvious!*
- *One final suggestion: a few deep breaths of fresh air can work wonders.*

ulcerative colitis (UC)

An inflammatory disease affecting the lining of the colon and rectum, ulcerative colitis causes pain, diarrhoea and the discharge of mucus and blood from the bowel.

HEALING FOODS

- *Ginger*
- *Turmeric*
- *Bread and other foods made with refined flour*
- *'Smoothies' and puréed soups*
- *Vegetables cooked until soft*

FOODS TO AVOID

- *During an acute attack the bowel needs to rest and no food should be taken. Follow medical advice.*
- *Reduce the residue in your diet. Avoid dried fruit, wholegrain products, brown rice, peas and beans, pulses, nuts and seeds, apples, sweetcorn and salad greens.*
- *Keep a food diary and look for 'triggers': milk, wheat and/or spicy foods, for example. Many sufferers of ulcerative colitis are lactose intolerant (see page 31).*

USEFUL RECIPES (WHEN THINGS ARE SETTLED)

Courgette and Mint Soup (page 106)
Pear Soup (see variations under Fruit Soup, page 109)
White Toast (topped with honey, crushed preserved ginger, roasted garlic or your favourite topping)

DID YOU KNOW?

- *Ulcerative colitis is a serious disease of Western cultures, and its prevalence is increasing. Estimates run as high as 100,000 sufferers in the UK. Women are more prone to this illness than men. Any age group can be affected, although people under the age of 35 are its most common victims.*
- *The cause of UC is unknown, although medical research indicates genetics may be a factor.*

vomiting

Vomiting is an involuntary act controlled by a centre in the brain, and has little to do with the stomach itself. It is often preceded by sweating, nausea, pallor and a slowed heartbeat.

HEALING FOODS

- *If you have a 'sensitive stomach', and frequently experience the unpleasantness of vomiting, try using more herbs and spices in your cooking. Good choices – in modest amounts – include mint, peppermint, garlic, dill, caraway, ginger, fennel, cardamom and cinnamon.*
- *Follow the BRAT diet during the acute phase of your illness (see page 26). When you are feeling better, add variety with any of the useful recipes below.*

FOODS TO AVOID

- *Food can upset your stomach if it is too fatty, contains too much chilli pepper, or is contaminated with dangerous bacteria. Food poisoning is the major cause of vomiting (see page 73).*
- *Too much alcohol.*

USEFUL RECIPES

Summer Berry Smoothie (page 218)
Ginger Milk Shake (page 220)
Stuffed Pears (page 98), substituting *Yoghurt Dressing* (page 162) for the mayonnaise used in the original recipe
Beetroot Soup (page 103)
Yoghurt Lemon Syllabub (page 184)
Waldorf Salad, using the variation made with apples and pears (page 99), substituting *Yoghurt Dressing* (page 162) for the mayonnaise used in the original recipe

DID YOU KNOW?

- *Vomiting is a symptom of a condition, and not a disorder in its own right. It usually occurs to rid the body of an unwanted substance. Causes include distension of the stomach by excess* food or drink, hormonal changes (as in pregnancy), infection of the gut (see 'Gastroenteritis'), toxins and poisonous substances, certain therapeutic treatments, and illnesses such as diabetes and encephalitis.

- *Medications may also cause stomach upset (see pages 226–30).*

- *Frequent or prolonged vomiting may indicate a serious underlying medical condition and should be discussed with your GP.*

WHEN YOU ARE ILL

- *Repeated vomiting changes your body chemistry. Be aware that when you vomit several times over a period of an hour or so, vital water, salt (sodium) and sugar are lost and need to be replaced. As soon as you feel able, sip a rehydration mixture made in the following way: boil 1 litre (1¾ pints) of water, add 1 teaspoon of table salt and 8 teaspoons of sugar. Stir and cool. (Rehydration mixtures can be purchased at a chemist, but this works just as well.)*

- *Four or five hours after your last episode of vomiting, try eating a small amount of mashed ripe banana. Bananas are an excellent source of energy, potassium and other minerals needed by your body. After that – and for the next several days – build up your strength on the BRAT diet, which consists of ripe bananas, rice, apples and toast (see pages 26–8).*

- *Vomiting is a common symptom of food poisoning caused by poor food hygiene (see pages 222–5).*

six marguerite patten's healthy gut recipes

cooking for invalids

Always follow the doctor's directions as to the type of food to be offered. If the doctor has not given specific instructions then read the advice in this book.

Pay particular attention to hygiene. This is always important, but people suffering from ill health are particularly vulnerable to infection. Utensils used for cooking and food preparation should be washed carefully. Keep separate chopping boards for cooked meat, raw meat and for other chopping purposes.

Choose cooking methods that make food easy to digest. Fried foods or rich dishes are not ideal for many gut ailments. Food should also be easy to eat, particularly if the person is confined to bed. Remove bones from poultry, game or meat joints and from fish. Cooked fruit, such as apricots, should have stones removed. Make sure portions are not too large. When someone is unwell and expending less physical energy, they do not need such large helpings of food. It is far better that they eat, and enjoy, a small meal rather than only part of a larger one.

Take a little time to make the dishes look, as well as taste, appetizing. Decorations or garnishes should be edible and chosen from the list of recommended ingredients. Colour plays a large part in making food attractive, so introduce naturally coloured ingredients where possible.

Make allowances for sick people being more difficult and fussy about food, especially if you are giving them new dishes. Some people will like to be consulted about their choice of menu, while others will find it troublesome and prefer the meal to be a surprise. Learn to understand the kind of person you are dealing with.

If a person is in bed, try to straighten the covers and sponge the patient's hands before serving a meal. Apart from being hygienic, this will freshen them and make them more inclined to anticipate their meal. Make sure that the tray is easy for them to support and that any plates or dishes are secure. Clear or thin soup may be easier to serve in a mug than in a soup bowl or plate.

Refreshing drinks, in covered jugs or a vacuum flask, should be left next to the bed. Change drinking water frequently. If a person is to be left for some time, provide them with a few biscuits, in an easy-to-open tin, and some fruit (if allowed) so they are not left feeling hungry. Do not leave partially eaten food in the room in the hope that it will be finished later. Apart from the fact that the patient is unlikely to do this, it is unhealthy, and food exposed to the air soon begins to look tired.

If you have to prepare food for yourself when you are far from well, try and do preparations early in the day or when you are feeling your best. Use simple cooking methods, such as in foil, so there is the minimum of clearing-up after the meal.

You should try and be as relaxed as possible before eating, so spoil yourself. Sit and enjoy a suitable drink, watch a light-hearted television programme or read part of an entertaining book or article.

cooking in foil

This is not only an easy way to cook food but also an excellent method of preserving flavour and reducing fat. It is particularly good for all kinds of fish and chicken portions.

Take large squares of thick foil (or a double thickness of thin foil). The squares must be sufficiently large to envelop each portion of food. Spread the centre of the foil with a few drops of oil.

Lay one fish or chicken portion in the centre of the foil. You can add spices and seasoning but be sparing as the flavour will be concentrated. You could add chopped herbs and/or finely chopped onion, slices of tomato, courgette (zucchini) or other vegetables or fruit below and above the fish or chicken. Remember that the additional ingredients must cook within the same time as the main food.

Top the fish or chicken with a few drops of oil and/or a small spoonful of wine, fruit juice or water. Seal the foil parcel(s) and place on a baking tray. Cook in a preheated oven set to 190°C/375°F/Gas Mark 5 (or 170–180°C with a fan oven). Fillets of fish take about 20 minutes, thicker cutlets 25–30 minutes and chicken 30–35 minutes.

Open the parcel(s) carefully because steam builds up inside the foil.

buying and using ingredients

As explained on page 93, it is advisable to buy organic ingredients when possible, as they are grown without the use of pesticides. When buying perishable ingredients, make sure they are fresh.

FISH, MEAT AND POULTRY

Check the date on the product and make sure these highly perishable foods are used well within that time. Store carefully in the refrigerator.

If minced meat is required, buy a portion of meat and mince this at home or chop it in a food processor. You can remove excess fat more easily and you know the meat is freshly minced or chopped. Minced or finely chopped meats deteriorate rapidly due to the many cut surfaces. The meat must be stored in the refrigerator and cooked as soon as possible after preparation. The cooked dish should be served soon after it is made or, when cold, stored in the freezer.

FRUIT AND VEGETABLES

Use fresh produce where possible or buy the frozen variety. If you have to purchase any canned fruit, choose the kind preserved in natural juice, rather than in syrup.

FRUIT DRINKS

Where possible, squeeze your own fruit to make sure the juice is as fresh and appetizing as possible. If buying fruit juices, check that they are made from whole, fresh fruit. Smoothies are an interesting way to enjoy fruit juices (*see page 218*).

HERBS

Various herbs are very important for a healthy gut (*see the list on pages 54–5*). The amounts of herbs given in the recipes are an essential contribution to a healthy diet. If possible, grow herbs in the garden or in a window box. Supermarkets and garden centres sell pots of herbs, which keep better than those in packs.

Any leftover herbs can be chopped and frozen. Parsley can be frozen in a bunch. When removed from the freezer it will be crisp, and you can crush it with your fingers. This must be done as soon as it is taken from the freezer or it will go limp.

SPICES

Dried spices deteriorate with storage so always buy them in small amounts. It is better to buy whole spices and grind them yourself so you enjoy the full flavour.

Ginger root is readily available. Freeze any leftover ginger or you could try planting it to grow your own ginger plant. Taken straight from the freezer, ginger is sufficiently hard to grate easily.

The amounts of spices given in the recipes are an essential contribution to a healthy diet.

OILS

Olive oil is very important for a healthy gut. Many of the following recipes specify 'extra virgin' or 'virgin' olive oil, which comes from the first pressing of the olives and is full of flavour. In other recipes that require less flavour, I have listed just 'olive oil'. Here a cheaper oil will suffice, but as you are aiming to heal the gut, you may decide to use the best oil at all times.

Always look for the term 'cold-pressed' on olive and other oils. The result is much better than when heat has been applied to extract the oil.

grains

Grains, other than wheat, are important for a healthy gut (*see pages 52–3*). Here are suggestions for ways in which they can be eaten.

BARLEY

This grain was used in the past far more than it is today. Pearl barley was added to stews to make them more sustaining and healthy. In the recipe section you will find a lamb dish in which pearl barley is an excellent addition (*page 126*). It is also given as an alternative to rice in the risotto on page 169.

Barley flour is not widely available, although health-food stores and supermarkets may stock it. You could use a small amount when making scones (*see page 204*).

BUCKWHEAT

In spite of its name, buckwheat is not a wheat but a member of the rhubarb family. It is gluten-free. Plain buckwheat is ground to make flour and is also sold as a hulled grain. Roasted buckwheat – the most popular form – is known as kasha. As this is pre-treated it does not need cooking. All you do is cover the grains with boiling water, leave until cold then strain them. The buckwheat is then ready to be part of a salad or to serve as a cold accompaniment to a main dish. It can be moistened with a dressing and mixed with grated raw carrots, cooked diced vegetables and chopped herbs.

To serve buckwheat hot: soften the grain, as in the directions above, and strain. Heat a little olive oil in a pan, add chopped onions and/or garlic, cook until soft then add the buckwheat and heat. Flavour with chopped herbs or with grated root ginger or chopped preserved ginger. This way of preparing buckwheat makes it an excellent part of a hot main dish.

MAIZE

This is the grain from which cornflour (cornstarch) is made. Corn in its various forms comes from maize, as do commercial cornflakes. Cornmeal is the fine form of maize used to make bread. This is often difficult to obtain in Britain, and polenta can be used instead.

MILLET

This grain is well known in many parts of the world but less so in Britain and America. It can take the place of oats in porridge. As it is a hard grain, it can be softened with water and allowed to stand for some hours before cooking it in a similar way to oatmeal or rolled oats.

OATS

Oats have been used for centuries to make porridge and, more recently, muesli (*see below*). A most adaptable grain, they give flavour to savoury and sweet dishes. Oats are a valuable source of soluble fibre and highly recommended for a healthy gut. Oatcakes are an excellent alternative to bread.

Porridge
In the past, porridge was made from medium and coarse oatmeal. This needed to be cooked for a long time in a saucepan or double saucepan. Nowadays, many people prefer speedy rolled oats, which make it quick and easy to cook porridge in individual bowls in the microwave.

Muesli
Although you can buy ready-prepared muesli, it is easy to make at home. You simply add your favourite ingredients to the oats, incorporating those recommended for a healthy gut (*see pages 54–5*). Mix a selection of chopped fresh fruit and dried fruit, such as dates, with nuts to the rolled oats; moisten with live yoghurt. If you prefer your muesli to be soft, prepare it the night before, cover and place in the refrigerator. You could toast the oats to give them more flavour, as in Cranachan (*see page 186*).

RICE

The importance of rice for a healthy gut is stressed on page 50. Choose brown rice if you are allowed as it has more flavour and extra nutrients. There are a number of savoury and sweet dishes based on rice in this book.

Rice noodles make a pleasant change from those based on wheat. Rice flour is an important ingredient in some biscuits and, like gluten-free flour, can take the place of wheat flour when making shortcrust pastry. Rice flour gives a crisp result but the pastry breaks easily and can be difficult to handle. The solution is to roll it between two sheets of clingfilm (saran wrap). Use the same proportion of fat to flour as in a standard shortcrust pastry recipe.

RYE

This grain, like barley, can be used to give new flavour to scones (*see page 204*). Rye bread and crispbread are readily available.

WHEAT

This is the most familiar grain. Most people enjoy wheat bread and foods based on wheat flour. Your gut trouble may mean you are advised to reduce your intake of wheat, or even to avoid eating it. There are alternatives (*see above*).

If you are intolerant to the gluten in wheat, remember that most types of pasta and couscous are prepared from this grain. Fortunately, you can obtain gluten-free pasta and there are rice noodles available. Rice or pearl barley can replace couscous.

GLUTEN CONTENT

Buckwheat, maize, millet and rice are free from gluten.

Milk

ᐰ

If you are intolerant to cow's milk, there are alternatives. Goat's milk is excellent, as is soya milk. You will find there are a number of other products made from both goat's and soya milk, including yoghurt.

Health-food stores sell milk alternatives such as almond milk, rice milk and sunflower seed milk. Coconut milk is a general favourite.

following the recipes

In most cases the recipes in this book are given in quantities for four people but they can easily be adapted for a smaller or larger household.

The dishes have been created to provide delicious ways to enjoy the healthy gut foods highlighted in Chapter 4. They are so appetizing and nutritious that everyone will enjoy and benefit from eating them. They are also simple to prepare. If you are unwell, you will need to conserve your energy. If you are caring for someone as well as for the rest of the family, your time will be at a premium.

Where a choice of ingredients is given, the ingredient mentioned first is the author's preference.

MEASUREMENTS

Ingredients in the recipes are given in metric, imperial and American measures so you can follow those with which you are most familiar.

Under American quantities, many ingredients are given in cup measures. This means using a true American cup. If using a metric or imperial cup, this is the equivalent of 230ml (8fl oz).

An American tablespoon is slightly smaller than a British one: 1¼ American tablespoons equal 1 British tablespoon. In recipes where only 1 tablespoon of an ingredient is given I have not changed the measure but 2 British tablespoons are shown as 2½ American ones.

When metric or imperial weights of ingredients are given in American cup measures, these vary enormously. For example, 115g (4oz) butter is equivalent to ½ an American cup, whereas 115g (4oz) flour is equivalent to 1 American cup.

INGREDIENTS

Use organic produce where possible. Make sure vegetables and fruit are fresh so that you obtain the maximum vitamin and mineral content.

Instructions about chopping, slicing, etc., are given in the recipes but it is assumed that vegetables and fruits are first washed then peeled if necessary.

Olive oil is used in some recipes. If the words 'virgin olive oil' are used, it means it is important for that particular dish. This top-grade oil is not essential where these words are not given.

TEMPERATURE

The oven temperatures are clearly given in the recipes. In the case of fan ovens, always check your manufacturer's instructions for there is a great difference in heat in these ovens. If worried, invest in an oven thermometer. You may find that cooking times are slightly reduced with a fan oven.

starters

 The following recipes are for simple dishes with which to start a meal. Starters should stimulate the appetite for the food that follows.

liver pâté SERVES 2–3

You can use calf's or lamb's liver for this pâté, the former having the more delicate flavour.
Whichever liver you choose, take care not to over-cook it. This basic recipe can be adapted in a
number of ways, as you will see in the 'Variations'. A generous amount of herbs is given in this first
version, as they are important for the diet.

Ingredients

METRIC (IMPERIAL)		AMERICAN
30g (1oz)	butter	2 tablespoons
1 tablespoon	olive oil	1 tablespoon
1	small onion, finely chopped	1
1	garlic clove, chopped	1
225g (8oz)	liver, thinly sliced	½lb
to taste	salt and freshly ground black pepper	to taste
1 teaspoon	English mustard (powder mixed with water or used from a tube) or Dijon mustard	1 teaspoon
2 teaspoons	chopped mint	2 teaspoons
3 teaspoons	chopped parsley	3 teaspoons
1½ tablespoons	live yoghurt	1¾ tablespoons

Method

1 Heat the butter with the oil in a good-sized frying pan. Add the onion and cook gently for 3 minutes, then put in the garlic and cook for a further 2 minutes. Move to the edge of the pan.

2 Add the liver to the pan and cook gently for about 1 minute; turn over and cook for the same time on the second side. (These times refer to cooking calf's liver; if using lamb's liver you may need to allow 1½–2 minutes on either side.) Remove the pan from the heat.

3 Add the rest of the ingredients, mixing with the liver. Transfer the mixture to a food processor or put in small batches in a liquidizer (blender) or through a mincer; process until you have a smooth pâté.

4 Place this into a container and cover at once, so the mixture does not become dry. Traditionally, pâtés are covered with melted butter, but it is important to avoid excess fat.

5   When cold, place the covered pâté in the refrigerator. Use within 2 days. Place portions of pâté on salad leaves and serve with toast.

Variations: add 30g–55g (1–2oz/¼–½ cup) chopped walnuts or blanched almonds to the smooth pâté after it has been liquidized or minced.

Chicken Liver Pâté: most chicken livers are obtainable in frozen form, so defrost then drain off any surplus moisture. Dry the livers well. To counteract their slightly bitter taste, put the dried livers into a bowl, cover with cold milk and leave for 4 hours. Drain and dry the livers again, then proceed as in the basic recipe or any of the variations that follow.

Fresh poultry livers should be sliced and cooked as in the basic recipe or any of the following variations.

Citrus Pâté: add 1–2 teaspoons finely grated lemon zest to the basic mixture; substitute chopped lemon balm leaves for the parsley but retain the mint.

Ginger Pâté: add 2 teaspoons grated or finely chopped root ginger to the pan and cook with the liver, and use ginger wine instead of the yoghurt. Instead of root ginger you can add 1–2 (2½) tablespoons finely chopped preserved ginger to the smooth pâté, after it has been liquidized or minced.

Sweet and Sour Pâté: instead of all yoghurt use ½ tablespoon balsamic vinegar, ½ tablespoon lemon juice and ½ (¾) tablespoon live yoghurt. Blend 4 (5) tablespoons finely chopped, dried, ready-to-eat apricots into the pâté after it has been liquidized or minced. Chopped, dried dessert dates could take the place of apricots or you could have a mixture of apricots and dates.

Freezing: these pâtés can be frozen for just one or two weeks. They lose texture if frozen for any longer.

hummus SERVES 4–6

There are literally dozens of different recipes for this savoury spread, based chiefly on chickpeas, garlic and sesame flavouring. This is my favourite version, but you could alter the proportions slightly. Hummus makes an excellent snack or hors d'oeuvre spread on toast, plain biscuits or with pitta bread.

Ingredients

METRIC (IMPERIAL)		AMERICAN
455g (1lb)	canned chickpeas	1lb
3 or to taste	garlic cloves, chopped	3 or to taste
1 tablespoon	lemon juice	1 tablespoon
1 tablespoon	sesame seed oil	1 tablespoon
few drops	extra virgin olive oil	few drops
1–2 tablespoons	sesame seeds	1–2½ tablespoons
to taste	sea salt and black or cayenne pepper	to taste

To garnish
chopped parsley
black and green olives

Method

1 Drain the chickpeas, rinse in cold water and dry. Put these with the other ingredients, except the garnish, into a liquidizer (blender) or food processor and make a smooth paste.
2 Spoon into a small dish and garnish.

Variations:

* *To use dried chickpeas, soak in a pan of cold water overnight, then put into fresh water, bring to simmering point and cook steadily for approximately 1½ hours or until tender, then drain.*
* *To make a softer paste, use more olive oil or a little live yoghurt.*
* *To give a stronger sesame flavour, either increase the amount of sesame seeds or mix with a little tahina paste (which you can buy).*

Freezing: not recommended.

stuffed pears SERVES 4

Pears, like apples, are not only ideal fruit for the diet but are also readily available throughout the year. In the following recipe, pears make an interesting and health-giving starter.

Ingredients

METRIC (IMPERIAL)		AMERICAN
2	large ripe firm pears	2
4 tablespoons	Vinaigrette Dressing (see *page 160*)	5 tablespoons
4 tablespoons	ricotta or other soft cheese	5 tablespoons
1–2 tablespoons	Mayonnaise (see *page 157*)	1–2½ tablespoons
4 tablespoons	chopped walnuts, pecan nuts or blanched almonds	5 tablespoons
2 tablespoons	chopped watercress leaves	2½ tablespoons

To garnish
watercress sprigs

Method

1   Halve then peel and core the pears. Place into the Vinaigrette Dressing immediately, so the fruit absorbs the flavour and keeps a good colour.

2   Mix the cheese, Mayonnaise, nuts and watercress leaves together and spoon into the cavity left by the cores.

3   Lift the pears from the dressing and place on the watercress sprigs, spooning any remaining dressing over the pears and watercress.

Variations: choose another cheese. A blue cheese, such as Stilton or Roquefort, can be mashed with the Mayonnaise to give a softer texture. If the pears are small, allow 1 whole fruit per person, slightly increasing the amounts in the filling, if necessary.

Freezing: not recommended.

waldorf salad SERVES 4

This popular, light, American dish is not only refreshing but also makes good use of ingredients recommended on the diet (see pages 54–5). The first recipe gives the classic ingredients, but under 'Variations' you will find other suggestions, which would make an equally appetizing start to a meal.

Ingredients

METRIC (IMPERIAL)		AMERICAN
I	celery heart, plus a few celery leaves	I
4	small-to-medium dessert apples	4
4 tablespoons	Mayonnaise (see *page 157*)	5 tablespoons
small bunch	grapes	small bunch
55g (2oz)	walnuts or pecan nuts, coarsely chopped	½ cup

Method

1 Cut the celery into neat, bite-sized pieces and select a few of the best celery leaves to garnish the salad.

2 The apples must be cored but the peel can be left on to give colour to the salad. If leaving the peel on, wash the apples thoroughly in cold water, then dry. Cut the fruit into neat dice and put into the Mayonnaise so it does not discolour.

3 If the grapes contain seeds, halve the fruit and gently pull out the seeds, trying to keep the grapes in a good shape. Mix with the celery, apples and dressing, then add the nuts. Spoon into one dish or individual dishes or glasses, and top with the celery leaves.

Variations:

- *Substitute diced melon for grapes.*
- *Make a lighter dressing by mixing 2 (2½) tablespoons Mayonnaise and 2–3 (2½–3¾) tablespoons live yoghurt together.*
- *Use thinly sliced chicory head(s) instead of celery.*
- *Instead of all apples use half apples and half diced, firm pears.*
- *Flavour the dressing with a little ground cinnamon or ginger.*

Freezing: not recommended.

soups

The soup recipes that follow are based on the foods recommended in the list of healthy gut foods in Chapter 4. Soups can be a start to a meal or they can be served as a complete light meal, followed by live yoghurt, fresh fruit or an interesting dessert. Spices and herbs enhance the flavour of the main ingredients in the soup. Never over-flavour a soup that is to precede a main course as it would spoil the palate for the dish to follow.

Stock is mentioned in the recipes. Where possible, prepare this yourself, as then you know that only fresh ingredients are used. If you have to rely on stock cubes or ready-prepared stock, be very fussy and choose the highest quality.

I have listed chicken stock first as this is very adaptable. Fish dishes, including fish soups, can be made with chicken stock. The choice of chicken stock seems to enhance the fish flavour.

chicken stock

These ingredients produce a mildly flavoured stock. For a stronger taste, simmer 1 or 2 uncooked chicken joints with the ingredients given below.

Use the carcass of a cooked chicken; break this into smaller pieces to enable more flavour to be extracted from the bones. Place the bones with 1 or 2 chopped onions, 1 or 2 sliced carrots and 1 or 2 chopped celery sticks into a good-sized saucepan, cover with water then add your chosen herbs, such as sprigs of tarragon, parsley and a little basil. It is better to add spices when you are making the individual soups. Season to taste. Place a tight-fitting lid on the pan and simmer gently for at least 1 hour.

If you are using the oven at a low setting, such as 140°C/275°F/Gas Mark 1 or 120–130°C with a fan-assisted oven, the stock could be prepared in a covered casserole. Allow at least 1½ hours' cooking time.

A pressure cooker is ideal for making stock. It takes only about 25–30 minutes at full pressure to achieve a good-flavoured liquid.

You can also use the microwave to make stock. Put the ingredients into a suitable dish, adding boiling water to save time. Cover and cook for ¾–1 hour on a third of the maximum output.

When the stock is ready, strain and cool it. Store for up to 2 days in the refrigerator or freeze in small containers.

beef stock

Follow the directions for chicken stock but use beef bones. Veal bones make a light-coloured stock very like chicken stock. Other meat bones could also be used.

fish stock

Use fish bones, skin and heads with the vegetables suggested under chicken stock. Fennel leaves and seeds or dill leaves are excellent flavourings. Add small pieces of lemon or lime zest to give a refreshing flavour.

Never simmer fish stock for too long as this spoils the flavour. In a saucepan, 20–25 minutes is quite sufficient, as is 10–15 minutes in a microwave.

vegetable stock

While you can use the liquid from cooking the vegetables of that day, you may find this lacks flavour. In this case, simmer the stock with chopped onion(s), carrot(s) and celery, as for chicken stock. Allow about 30 minutes in a saucepan or 15 minutes in the microwave. Fresh mint or tarragon are excellent herbs to enhance the taste of a vegetable stock.

Freezing: remove as much fat as possible and freeze in small containers.

beetroot (beet) soup SERVES 4

Most people enjoy the sweet flavour of beetroot, and the vegetable makes an excellent soup. Cooked beetroot(s) are the basis of this recipe. Choose the small ones as they have the most appealing taste. This soup is equally good cold or hot. If you want to serve the soup without sieving or liquidizing (blending) it then finely chop or grate the ingredients. These can be roughly diced if you are going to produce a smooth soup by sieving or liquidizing.

Ingredients

METRIC (IMPERIAL)		AMERICAN
I tablespoon	olive oil	I tablespoon
I	medium onion, chopped	I
I	garlic clove, chopped	I
I	medium carrot, chopped	I
340g (12oz)	cooked beetroot, weight when skinned	¾lb
850ml (1½ pints)	vegetable or chicken stock	3¾ cups
½ teaspoon	ground cinnamon	½ teaspoon
to taste	sea salt and freshly ground black pepper	to taste
1–2 teaspoons	caraway seeds	1–2 teaspoons
140–285ml (¼ to ½ pint)	live yoghurt	⅔–1⅓ cups

To garnish
chopped coriander (cilantro) or parsley

Method

1 Heat the oil in a large saucepan. Add the onion and cook gently for 5 minutes. Add the garlic and the carrots and cook for a further 5 minutes. Stir well during this time so the vegetables do not discolour.

2 Add all the other ingredients except the yoghurt and the garnish. Simmer for 10 minutes.

3 **To serve hot**: without liquidizing, simply stir the required amount of yoghurt into the hot mixture and heat carefully. After liquidizing, return the ingredients to the pan, add the amount of yoghurt required and heat without boiling. Garnish and serve.
   To serve cold: chill the soup well, either with or without liquidizing. Top with the yoghurt and garnish.

Freezing: the soup freezes well without the yoghurt. Add this when defrosted.

celery soup SERVES 4–5

Celery is a valuable vegetable for a healthy gut and makes an interesting soup. You may find that after liquidizing (blending) the ingredients you still have some rather stringy pieces of celery. If so, rub them through a sieve for a smooth soup. You can avoid this if you trim the string-like parts from the outer celery leaves before cooking. Include some celery leaves for colour and flavour.

Ingredients

METRIC (IMPERIAL)		AMERICAN
2 tablespoons	olive oil	2½ tablespoons
I	medium head of celery, chopped	I
2	small onions, chopped	2
2	small leeks, sliced	2
2	small potatoes, diced	2
I litre (1¾ pints)	chicken stock or water	scant 4½ cups
1–1½ teaspoons	grated nutmeg	1–1½ teaspoons
140ml (¼ pint)	live yoghurt	⅔ cup
to taste	sea salt, freshly ground white pepper	to taste

To garnish
celery leaves and paprika

Method

1 Heat the oil in a saucepan and add the celery, onions and leeks. Turn the vegetables in the oil until well coated, lower the heat and cook gently for 6 minutes, stirring from time to time.

2 Add the potatoes with the stock or water and the nutmeg. Bring just to simmering then cover the saucepan and cook for 15–20 minutes or until all the vegetables are tender. Liquidize (blend) until smooth and return to the pan.

3 Pour in the yoghurt then assess the consistency. This should be a thick soup, but if it is too thick add a little more stock, water or yoghurt. Taste and adjust the seasoning. Heat without boiling, garnish and serve.

Celery and Apple Soup: omit onions and use 2 small peeled and diced dessert apples.

Freezing: the soup freezes well without the yoghurt. Add this when defrosted.

cheese soup SERVES 4

People who are unwell may not be tempted by cheese and biscuits or bread so it is good to provide the protein value of cheese in a soup. The vegetables, herbs and spices add interest and nutrients.

Ingredients

METRIC (IMPERIAL)		AMERICAN
225g (8oz)	cheese, preferably Cheddar, see stage 1	½lb
1 tablespoon	virgin olive oil	1 tablespoon
2	small shallots/1 small onion, finely chopped	2
1	garlic clove, finely chopped	1
570ml (1 pint)	vegetable or chicken stock	2½ cups
2	medium carrots, finely chopped or grated	2
3 tablespoons	fresh or frozen peas	scant 4 tablespoons
3 tablespoons	celery heart, finely chopped	scant 4 tablespoons
to taste	sea salt and freshly ground white pepper	to taste
½–1 teaspoon	ground cinnamon	½–1 teaspoon
230ml (8fl oz)	milk/soya milk/rice milk	1 cup
2 level teaspoons	cornflour (cornstarch)	2 level teaspoons
1–2 tablespoons	chopped mint	1–2½ tablepoons

Method

1 Grate the cheese if suitable or divide into small portions so it will dissolve rapidly.

2 Heat the oil in a saucepan. Add the shallots or onion and cook gently for 3 minutes, then stir in the garlic and cook for a further minute.

3 Pour in the stock and bring to the boil, then add the vegetables with a little seasoning and the cinnamon. Cover the pan and cook fairly briskly for about 7 minutes or until the vegetables are just tender but not overcooked.

4 Blend the milk and cornflour, and stir into the soup until thick. Add the cheese and mint and heat only until the cheese has dissolved. Season and serve.

Rice and Cheese Soup: increase the amount of stock by 140ml (¼ pint/⅔ cup), bring to the boil as stage 3, stir in 2 (2½) level tablespoons long-grain rice and simmer for about 6 minutes, then add the vegetables and continue as the recipe above.

Freezing: this is best eaten when freshly made.

courgette (zucchini) and mint soup

SERVES 4

While this soup can be served hot, I prefer it well chilled. It is most refreshing on a hot summer's day. There is no need to peel the courgettes; simply cut away the firm ends and wash them well.

Ingredients

METRIC (IMPERIAL)		AMERICAN
1 tablespoon	light olive oil	1 tablespoon
2	shallots, chopped	2
340g (12oz)	courgettes, thinly sliced	¾lb
3 tablespoons	vegetable stock or water	scant 4 tablespoons
2–3 tablespoons	mint leaves	2½–3¾ tablespoons
570ml (1 pint)	low-fat live yoghurt	2½ cups
to taste	sea salt and freshly ground black pepper	to taste
1–2 teaspoons	cumin or sesame seeds	1–2 teaspoons

To garnish

chopped mint

Method

1 Heat the oil, add the shallots and cook very gently for 5 minutes. Do not allow them to darken. Put in the courgettes and the stock or water.

2 Simmer for about 6 minutes or until the courgettes are tender, stirring well during this time. Allow the mixture to become cold.

3 Put all the ingredients into a liquidizer (blender) or food processor and whiz until you have a smooth purée. Chill well and top with the mint just before serving.

Variations:

* *Other vegetables can be served in the same way, e.g. sliced cooked cucumber (if allowed on the diet), florets of cauliflower or broccoli.*
* *Use half yoghurt and half milk or half yoghurt and half apple juice (unsweetened if possible).*
* *Add 1–2 teaspoons of mild curry powder or paste to the courgettes at the end of stage 1.*

Freezing: freeze the cooked purée without the yoghurt, to be added when defrosted.

chicken and almond soup SERVES 4–5

The idea of thickening liquids with almonds, rather than flour or cornflour (cornstarch), is not a new one. Almonds have been used for culinary purposes for centuries and are an important ingredient for a healthy gut.

Ground almonds are given in the following recipe but you could blanch (skin) and chop whole almonds in a liquidizer (blender) or food processor. It is important to use a strongly flavoured chicken stock (see page 101). To add extra food value and flavour, a chicken breast and a small amount of rice are simmered in the stock.

Ingredients

METRIC (IMPERIAL)		AMERICAN
I litre (1¾ pints)	chicken stock	scant 4½ cups
I small	onion, left whole	I small
I tablespoon	long-grain white rice	I tablespoon
I teaspoon	finely grated lemon zest	I teaspoon
I sprig	tarragon	I sprig
I	chicken breast, skinned	I
55g (2oz)	ground almonds	½ cup
to taste	sea salt and freshly ground white pepper	to taste
to taste	lemon juice	to taste

To garnish
live yoghurt
chopped tarragon

Method

1 Put the stock and onion into a saucepan, bring just to boiling point then add the rice, lemon zest, tarragon and chicken breast.
2 Cover the saucepan and simmer for 15 minutes or until the rice is cooked and the chicken is tender. Remove the chicken breast and chop it finely.
3 Discard the onion and sprig of tarragon, stir the ground almonds into the soup, season to taste and add a little lemon juice. Return the chicken breast to the pan and heat the soup for 2 minutes. Serve topped with the yoghurt and tarragon.

Freezing: this soup freezes well.

fruit soups

Some people might think a fruit soup sounds rather unusual, but when you have tasted one you will be completely converted. Although fruit soups are generally served well chilled, they are delicious warm, or even piping hot. When making a fruit soup, remember it is a soup and not to be confused with a smoothie (*see page 218*), so it should not be too sweet. In many recipes wine or water is used as the liquid, but in the fruit soup recipes I have suggested using a certain amount of stock. In the case of gut problems the soup should help stimulate the appetite. Even a little seasoning could be added to make the dish a suitable first course or light main dish. Mango Soup is a favourite of mine. Other, more everyday fruit soups are just as pleasant (*see 'Variations'*).

mango soup SERVES 4

Ingredients

METRIC (IMPERIAL)		AMERICAN
140ml (¼ pint)	mild-flavoured chicken or vegetable stock	⅔ cup
1 medium	shallot, left whole	1
2 medium	mangoes, fully ripe	2
1–2 tablespoons	lemon or lime juice	1–2½ tablespoons
285ml (½ pint)	dry white wine or cider or water with	1⅓ cups
	1 tablespoon extra lemon juice	
very little	sea salt and ground white pepper, optional	very little
1 teaspoon	ground cinnamon	1 teaspoon
140 ml (¼ pint)	live yoghurt or crème fraîche	⅔ cup

To garnish
raspberries or strawberry slices
live yoghurt or crème fraîche
mint leaves

Method

1   Bring the stock to the boil, add the shallot and the mango flesh. You need to cut away the skin and scoop all the flesh from both sides of the large stones. Simmer for 3 minutes only, then remove and discard the shallot.

2 Add all the other ingredients, except the yoghurt or crème fraîche, and heat for 3 minutes only. Cool and liquidize (blend) until a smooth purée.

3 Add the yoghurt or crème fraîche and liquidize again. If slightly too thick, add a little more yoghurt. Chill well and serve topped with a few summer berries, yoghurt or crème fraîche and mint leaves.

Variations: to serve hot, heat in a saucepan, in the top of a double pan or in a basin in the microwave. Serve topped with small, crisp croutons.

Apple Soup

Use 340g/¾lb peeled and sliced cooking apples, or a mixture of cooking and dessert apples (Cox's or another type that cooks well). Simmer in the stock as stage 1 above, until the fruit is very soft. Continue as the recipe – the shallot can be liquidized (blended) with the other ingredients to give a more savoury taste. Replace the ground cinnamon with ground ginger. Garnish with a little sliced preserved ginger as well as yoghurt or crème fraîche and mint.

Banana Soup

Simmer the shallot as stage 1, remove this and add 3 skinned medium bananas, cut into thin slices. Heat for 2 minutes only, then continue as the recipe. The spices can be replaced by 1–2 teaspoons grated lemon or lime zest.

Peach or Nectarine Soup

Use about 4 medium-sized, ripe fruit. Skin them by lowering into boiling water for 30 seconds, then plunging into cold water, pulling away the skin. Slice the fruit and discard the stones. Continue as the recipe above. Ground cinnamon blends well with these fruits, or use 1–2 teaspoons lemon or lime zest instead.

Pear Soup

This makes an excellent hot or cold soup. Follow the recipe for Apple Soup but choose ripe Conference or Comice pears, or good dessert pears. Use 1 tablespoon lemon or lime juice and 2 (2½) tablespoons orange juice. Flavour with ground cinnamon or ground ginger. Top with mint leaves and twists of lemon or lime and orange zest.

Freezing: these soups can be frozen, preferably without the yoghurt, which can be added when they are defrosted. However, they are better freshly made.

lentil soup SERVES 4

Lentils are a good source of protein, so this soup could be served as a light main dish. Smaller portions would make an excellent first course. I prefer to use orange/red lentils for this soup, rather than the more expensive French Puy type, because they give the soup a most tempting colour. Traditionally, lentil soup is often made with the stock from boiling bacon or ham but, if you use vegetable stock, it is suitable for vegetarians. The additional vegetables, with the ginger, cumin and herbs, add to the health-giving properties of this soup. If you prefer to serve the soup without liquidizing (blending) it then the vegetables must be chopped finely and evenly.

Ingredients

METRIC (IMPERIAL)		AMERICAN
2 tablespoons	olive oil	2½ tablespoons
2	medium onions, chopped	2
1–2	garlic cloves, chopped	1–2
2	medium carrots, chopped	2
2–3	celery sticks, chopped	2–3
1	medium dessert apple, peeled, cored and chopped	1
850ml (1½ pints)	bacon or vegetable stock	3¾ cups
140g (5oz)	lentils, rinsed in cold water and drained	⅝ cup
½ teaspoon	ground cumin	½ teaspoon
1 tablespoon	ground root ginger	1 tablespoon
½–1 tablespoon	lime juice	½–1 tablespoon
2 teaspoons	chopped basil	2 teaspoons
2 teaspoons	chopped parsley	2 teaspoons
to taste	sea salt and freshly ground black pepper	to taste
140ml (¼ pint)	milk	⅔ cup
	To garnish	
140ml (¼ pint)	live yoghurt	⅔ cup
	chopped basil	
	chopped parsley	

Method

1   Heat the oil in a large saucepan, add all the vegetables and the apple and turn in the oil for 2 minutes. Pour in the stock, bring this to the boil then add the lentils and the rest of the ingredients except the milk.

2   Bring to simmering point, cover the pan and cook gently for 30–35 minutes until the ingredients are tender, then add the milk and reheat. Garnish and serve.

Variation: add the milk to the hot soup and liquidize (blend). Either reheat or chill well. (The smooth version of the soup is excellent cold.)

Freezing: this soup freezes well. Add the garnish when the soup is defrosted and ready to serve.

oatmeal and watercress soup SERVES 4–6

Oatmeal and watercress are appetizing and useful ingredients for a healthy gut. Together they make an interesting and unusual soup. While fine oatmeal gives a smoother texture, rolled oats could be substituted.

Ingredients

METRIC (IMPERIAL)		AMERICAN
1 tablespoon	olive oil	1 tablespoon
2	medium onions, finely chopped	2
2 tablespoons	medium or fine oatmeal	2½ tablespoons
570ml (1 pint)	vegetable or chicken stock	2½ cups
2	medium carrots, finely chopped	2
285ml (½ pint)	milk	1⅓ cups
to taste	sea salt and freshly ground black pepper	to taste
140ml (¼ pint)	live yoghurt	⅔ cup
55g (2oz)	watercress leaves, chopped	1 cup

To garnish

small watercress leaves

Method

1 Heat the oil in a saucepan, add the onions and cook gently for 5 minutes. Add the oatmeal and blend with the onions.
2 Pour in the stock and bring just to simmering point, stirring well to mix with the oatmeal and onions. Tip in the carrots. Cover the pan and simmer gently for 20 minutes, stirring from time to time.
3 Add the milk and seasoning, and simmer for a further 10 minutes.
4 Finally add the yoghurt and chopped watercress and heat for 5 minutes. Adjust the seasoning and serve topped with more watercress.

Variation: sieve or liquidize (blend) the soup before adding the yoghurt and chopped watercress. Return the smooth soup to the pan then stir in these ingredients and heat.

Freezing: the smooth soup (as described under Variation) freezes best. Add the yoghurt and watercress after defrosting.

salmon broth

This soup is full of colour and interest, and there is no need for sieving or liquidizing (blending). I have chosen salmon because it is colourful and popular. Other fish could be used instead, preferably cold-water fish rich in health-giving essential fatty acids. Other fish in this group are trout, herrings and sardines.

Ingredients

METRIC (IMPERIAL)		AMERICAN
455g (1lb)	salmon fillet	1lb
570ml (1 pint)	fish or chicken stock	2½ cups
85g (3oz)	long-grain rice	½ cup
to taste	salt and freshly ground white pepper	to taste
2 tablespoons	finely diced fennel root	2½ tablespoons
2 tablespoons	finely diced carrots	2½ tablespoons
285ml (½ pint)	milk	1⅓ cups
2 teaspoons	chopped fennel leaves	2 teaspoons

To garnish

single cream or live yoghurt

chopped parsley and fennel leaves

Method

1   Remove the skin from the fish and check there are no small bones. Cut the flesh into 1.25cm (½-inch) pieces.

2   Pour the stock into a saucepan, stir in the rice with the seasoning and simmer for 10 minutes. Add the fennel root and carrots and continue simmering for another 5 minutes or until the rice is nearly cooked.

3   Add the milk, fennel leaves and fish. Cook for a further 5 minutes or until both rice and fish are ready to serve. Top with the cream or yoghurt and the herbs.

Freezing: not recommended as the ingredients tend to become over-soft.

fish dishes

Fish is an important part of any healthy diet. When combined with other healing ingredients, it makes a good food for people concerned about their digestive health. You will see that the recipes I have chosen here feature fish but also incorporate many of the foods discussed in Chapter 4. Some of these additional ingredients may seem unusual with fish but do not worry – the dishes have been tested carefully and the extra items add interest as well as nutritional value.

In all the recipes you could choose a different kind of fish to the one recommended, although I have selected the fish I think is best. However, it is advisable to use oily fish as often as possible.

potted salmon

This is an ideal way of serving fish for a light snack. It is equally good on hot toast or with a salad. Virgin olive oil has replaced the usual butter, so you produce a softer texture than usual. Cumin, dill and cinnamon (all important in the diet) are added to the fish.

Ingredients

METRIC (IMPERIAL)		AMERICAN
340g (12oz)	cooked salmon	¾lb
2 tablespoons	virgin olive oil	2½ tablespoons
½–1 teaspoon	ground cumin	½–1 teaspoon
1–2 teaspoons	chopped dill leaves	1–2 teaspoons
½ teaspoon	ground cinnamon	½ teaspoon
to taste	sea salt and freshly ground black pepper	to taste

Method

1 Break the salmon into very fine flakes, discarding all bones or skin. If flaking the fish in a food processor, take great care not to over-process as this makes the fish sticky.

2 Add all the other ingredients and mix gently but thoroughly. Put into one or more small containers and cover with foil. Store in the refrigerator for up to 2 days.

Variation: instead of oil use up to 85g (3oz) of melted unsalted butter. You could cover the potted salmon with a layer of melted butter too.

Freezing: not recommended.

moroccan fish with dates SERVES 4–6

Cooking fish with dates may sound strange but it is a delightful combination of flavours. I first tasted this dish in Tangier many years ago and it has since become a family favourite. Dates are included in the list of important foods on pages 54–5, as are rice, ginger and cinnamon. White fish is recommended here but this could be replaced by oily trout. Ask the fishmonger to remove the head and backbone from the fish. These could be used to make fish stock (see page 102).

Ingredients

METRIC (IMPERIAL)		AMERICAN
55g (2oz)	long-grain rice	⅓ cup
¼ teaspoon	salt	¼ teaspoon
225g (8oz)	dried dessert dates (stoned weight)	½lb
55g (2oz)	almonds, blanched and chopped	½ cup
½ teaspoon (see stage 2)	ground ginger	½ teaspoon (see stage 2)
½ teaspoon (see stage 2)	ground cinnamon	½ teaspoon (see stage 2)
85g (3oz)	butter, melted	⅜ cup
shake	freshly ground black pepper	shake
140ml (¼ pint)	fish stock or water	⅔ cup
1 medium	onion, finely chopped	1 medium
900g (2lb)	whole codling or haddock (boned weight)	2lb

Method

1 Cook the rice in boiling, salted water until just softened. Drain well.

2 Cut the stoned dates into long matchsticks and mix with the rice, almonds and most of the ginger and cinnamon. Save a little of the spices for the cooking liquid. Add just over half the butter and the pepper.

3 Preheat the oven to 180°C/350°F/Gas Mark 4 or 160–170°C with a fan oven. Use a little of the remaining butter to grease a large casserole, then add the fish stock or water, the onion and remaining spices.

4 Insert the rice and date mixture into the fish, and tie or secure with fine skewers. Place in the casserole and top with the last of the butter. Do not cover the casserole. Bake for 40–45 minutes. Serve with a green vegetable or salad.

Variations:

If more convenient, stuff individual small-boned fish and bake for about 25 minutes. Olive oil could be used instead of butter.

Freezing: do not freeze the cooked dish. Defrosted and well-dried uncooked fish could be used.

roast fish with herb sauce SERVES 4

Most white fish, as well as salmon, is suitable for this dish. Buy fairly thick cutlets. The fish acquires a pleasing golden-brown colour, making it very inviting. You could alter the suggested herbs for the sauce to suit your own preferences.

Ingredients

METRIC (IMPERIAL)		AMERICAN
2 tablespoons	olive oil	2½ tablespoons
4	cutlets white fish or salmon	4
1 teaspoon	finely grated lemon or lime zest	1 teaspoon
to taste	sea salt and freshly ground black pepper	to taste
	For the sauce	
2 tablespoons	finely chopped parsley	2½ tablespoons
1 tablespoon	finely chopped fennel or dill leaves	1 tablespoon
1–2 teaspoons	finely chopped basil leaves	1–2 teaspoons
1 teaspoon	finely grated lemon or lime zest	1 teaspoon
1 tablespoon	lemon or lime juice	1 tablespoon
1 tablespoon	extra virgin olive oil	1 tablespoon

Method

1 Preheat the oven to 190°C/375°F/Gas Mark 5 or 170–180°C with a fan oven.
2 Brush the base of the roasting tin (pan) or dish with a little of the oil, put in the fish and top with the rest of the oil and zest. Season lightly. Do not cover the dish. Roast for 15–20 minutes or until the fish is just cooked, taking care not to overcook.
3 Meanwhile mix together all the ingredients for the sauce. Season to taste and spoon over the fish immediately before serving. Serve with a mixture of cooked vegetables.

Freezing: do not freeze the cooked fish, but defrosted frozen fish could be used. Dry this well before cooking.

salmon with grapes SERVES 4

This dish has an interesting mixture of flavours. The wine and grapes give a refreshing touch to the fish. The horseradish blends extremely well with salmon and has a piquant flavour. Use fresh horseradish if possible but horseradish cream could be substituted (see 'Variations').

Ingredients

METRIC (IMPERIAL)		AMERICAN
4	salmon cutlets	4
285ml (½ pint)	dry white wine	1⅓ cups
2	fairly large mint sprigs	2
1 tablespoon	grated horseradish or to taste	1 tablespoon
to taste	sea salt and freshly ground black pepper	to taste
115g (4oz)	grapes, preferably seedless	¼lb
2 tablespoons	pine kernels	2½ tablespoons

To garnish
chopped mint

Method

1 Preheat the oven to 190°C/375°F/Gas Mark 5 or 170–180°C with a fan oven. Put the salmon cutlets into a large casserole.

2 Add the wine. Bruise the mint leaves with a rolling pin so the maximum flavour is extracted, then add to the fish with the horseradish, seasoning and grapes. If the grapes contain seeds, split them with the point of a small knife and pull out the seeds.

3 Cover the casserole and bake for 25–30 minutes. Add the pine kernels towards the end of the cooking so they retain their firm texture. Remove the mint sprigs before serving but top with freshly chopped mint. Cauliflower and saba (buckwheat) noodles are excellent accompaniments.

Variations:
Use 2 (2½) tablespoons horseradish cream instead of grated horseradish.
Use salmon fillets, reducing the cooking time by a few minutes.

Freezing: do not freeze the cooked dish. Frozen salmon could be used.

scottish herrings SERVES 4

This is an old, traditional fish dish in which boned herrings are coated with oatmeal then cooked. As frying is not an ideal method of cooking, bake the fish in the oven or cook them in salt (see 'Variation').

If the fishmonger has not boned the fish you will find this quite easy to do (see stage 1 below).

Ingredients

METRIC (IMPERIAL)		AMERICAN
4	large fresh herrings	4
2 tablespoons	milk or yoghurt	2½ tablespoons
40g (1½oz)	fine or medium oatmeal	scant ½ cup
to taste	sea salt and freshly ground black pepper	to taste
1 tablespoon	olive oil	1 tablespoon

To garnish
lemon wedges

Method

1   To bone the herrings: slit the fish along the stomachs. Carefully remove the intestines and discard them, except for the roes which can be coated with oatmeal and cooked with the boned fish. Cut off the heads, then turn each fish over so the skin side is uppermost. Place on a firm chopping board. Rub your forefinger very firmly down the centre of each fish. Turn the fish over and you will find you can remove the backbones and nearly all the smaller bones. Any odd bones remaining can be pulled out with tweezers or your fingers.

2   Wash the fish in cold water and dry thoroughly, then brush with the milk or yoghurt and coat on both sides with the oatmeal, seasoned with the salt and pepper. Do the same with the roes. If time permits, leave in the refrigerator for 30 minutes before cooking so the coating sets on the fish.

3   Preheat the oven to 200°C/400°F/Gas Mark 6 or 180–190°C with a fan oven. Brush a large, flat tin or ovenproof dish with a little of the oil. Preheat this for 3 minutes (to stop the fish sticking) then place the fish on the heated tin or dish, preferably in a completely flat layer.

4   Dribble the remaining oil over the top of the fish and bake for 25 minutes. The roes cook more quickly so should be added to the tin or dish after 10 minutes. Garnish and serve.

Variation: the truly Scottish way of cooking herrings is to fill a large frying pan with a thin layer of salt. Heat the salt for 3–4 minutes, add the fish and cook for 5 minutes on each side. The roes take about 3 minutes on either side.

Freezing: the cooked fish are spoiled by freezing but you could use defrosted herrings. Dry well once thawed.

trout with walnuts and ginger wine

SERVES 4

Trout, like salmon, are members of the oily fish group and an ideal food for everyone. The addition of walnuts and mellow ginger wine gives the fish a wonderful flavour, and both ingredients help promote a healthy gut. If you are fortunate enough to have fresh walnuts, skin them before using. The fish can be poached or baked; both methods are given below.

Ingredients

METRIC (IMPERIAL)		AMERICAN
4	rainbow or salmon trout	4
to taste	salt and freshly ground black pepper	to taste
170ml (6fl oz)	ginger wine	⅔ cup
115ml (4fl oz)	fish stock or water	½ cup
2 teaspoons	chopped tarragon leaves or ½ teaspoon dried tarragon	2 teaspoons
2 teaspoons	grated root ginger	2 teaspoons
85g (3oz)	walnuts, coarsely chopped	¾ cup
	To garnish	
	tarragon or parsley sprigs	
	lime or lemon wedges	

Method

1 Split the fish and remove the intestines. The heads should be cut off too, although these are left on in many trout dishes. Season the fish lightly.

2 **To steam the fish**: pour the wine and stock or water into a fish kettle or large saucepan. Add the tarragon, ginger, then the fish and walnuts. Cover the fish kettle or saucepan to retain the moisture and cook for 10–12 minutes. During this time the liquid can be spooned over the fish once or twice.

To bake the fish: preheat oven to 190°C/375°F/Gas Mark 5 or 170–180°C with a fan oven. Put all ingredients into a large casserole, cover tightly and bake for 30 minutes.

3 Garnish and serve. Cooked rice/rice noodles and carrots are ideal accompaniments.

Freezing: do not freeze the cooked fish; defrosted frozen trout could be used.

meat, poultry and game

You can use your usual, preferred cooking methods for most of the recipes in this chapter. With a little imagination, your favourite recipes can be adapted to include foods that are particularly beneficial for a healthy gut. Boosting the amount of fruits, vegetables, herbs and spices in your cooking can play a big part in helping to control a gut disorder. You could add a little ginger or horseradish to a stuffing or gravy, or make meats and poultry more interesting with some of the important fruits.

beef with pineapple and ginger

In this simple stir-fry, the beef is flavoured with fresh pineapple and ginger. If using the tender steaks given, the marinade is not essential to tenderize the meat, but it does impart an excellent flavour. If using more economical beef, as suggested under 'Variations', then the marinade plays a large part in making the meat beautifully tender.

Ingredients

METRIC (IMPERIAL)		AMERICAN
4	steaks, either fillet or rump	4
	Marinade	
I tablespoon	olive or sunflower oil	I tablespoon
2 tablespoons	rice vinegar or dry sherry	2½ tablespoons
2	garlic cloves, finely chopped	2
2 teaspoons	root ginger, finely grated	2 teaspoons
	For stir-frying	
225g (8oz)	fresh pineapple (skinned weight)	½lb
I	red pepper, deseeded	I
I tablespoon	olive or sunflower oil	I tablespoon
about 12	spring onions (scallions), thinly sliced	about 12
140ml (¼ pint)	beef or chicken stock	⅔ cup
I tablespoon	lemon juice	I tablespoon
I tablespoon	honey	I tablespoon
I teaspoon	cornflour (cornstarch)	I teaspoon
to taste	salt and freshly ground black pepper	to taste

Method

1 Cut the steak into neat fingers. Mix the ingredients for the marinade together in a shallow dish and add the steak. Turn around in the marinade until covered and leave for about 15 minutes.

2 Cut the pineapple and the red pepper into thin strips.

3 Heat the oil in a wok or large frying pan (skillet), add the spring onions (scallions) and stir-fry for 2 minutes. Add the meat and the marinade together with the pineapple and pepper. Continue stir-frying until the meat is tender.

4   Blend the stock, lemon juice, honey and cornflour. Add to the pan and stir-fry until you have a thin sauce.

5   Season to taste and serve with cooked rice or rice noodles and a green vegetable.

Variations:

* *Use best-quality topside of beef and allow about 30 minutes in the marinade.*
* *Adapt this dish with slices of chicken, turkey or lean pork.*
* *To give more flavour, add 1 tablespoon of soya sauce to the stock at stage 4.*

Freezing: do not freeze. Defrosted and well-dried frozen meat could be used.

lamb with barley and caper sauce SERVES 4

In this recipe the less expensive part of lamb is cooked with a selection of mixed root vegetables and pearl barley. The dish is served with Caper Sauce. If you are anxious to avoid any extra fat, cook the dish a day in advance, allow it to become quite cold and place in the refrigerator until the next day. You can then lift off and discard any solid fat that has formed on the top of the stew before reheating.

Ingredients

METRIC (IMPERIAL)		AMERICAN
85g (3oz)	pearl barley	⅜ cup
as required	water	as required
1kg (2¼lb)	middle neck of lamb, jointed	2¼lb
to taste	sea salt and freshly ground black pepper	to taste
few	sprigs of mint	few
455g (1lb)	mixed vegetables, e.g. carrots, turnip, celery, parsnip, swede	1lb
	Caper Sauce	
30g (1oz)	butter or margarine	2 tablespoons
30g (1oz)	plain (all-purpose) flour	¼ cup
285ml (½ pint)	milk	1⅓ cups
140ml (¼ pint)	lamb stock, see stage 5	⅔ cup
3 teaspoons	capers	3 teaspoons
	To garnish	
	chopped mint	

Method

1 Put the pearl barley into a saucepan with cold water, bring to the boil, strain and discard the liquid.
2 Put the lamb into a large saucepan with water to cover. Add a little seasoning and the mint. Bring to simmering point and simmer for 20 minutes.
3 Cut the vegetables into fairly large pieces (if small they can be left whole). Add to the pan with the pearl barley. Check there is plenty of liquid. Tightly cover the saucepan and simmer for 1 hour or until the meat is tender.

4 **Caper Sauce**: when the lamb is nearly cooked, prepare the sauce. Melt the butter or margarine in a small saucepan, stir in the flour then add the milk. Stir or whisk as the sauce comes to the boil and thickens.

5 Spoon out 140ml (¼ pint/⅔ cup) of stock from cooking the lamb and whisk into the sauce. Add the capers and season to taste.

6 Remove the sprigs of mint from the stew. Lift the lamb, barley and vegetables onto the serving dish with a large ladle. Top with the chopped mint. Pour the Caper Sauce into a sauceboat. Serve with Brussels sprouts or cauliflower.

Freezing: the stew can be frozen but the vegetables tend to lose their texture.

lamb with pears and pine nuts SERVES 4

Pears can enhance the flavour of meat dishes, such as in this recipe. They are an important fruit for a healthy gut.

Ingredients

METRIC (IMPERIAL)		AMERICAN
2	large, firm and almost ripe pears, peeled, cored and thickly sliced	2
225ml (7½fl oz)	white wine	scant 1 cup
1 teaspoon	balsamic or sherry vinegar	1 teaspoon
2 teaspoons	chopped tarragon leaves	2 teaspoons
1 tablespoon	olive oil	1 tablespoon
2 tablespoons	finely chopped spring onions (scallions)	2½ tablespoons
4	lean lamb chops or fillets	4
to taste	salt and freshly ground black pepper	to taste

To garnish

sliced pine nuts

mint leaves

Method

1 Place the sliced pears in the wine so they do not discolour, add the vinegar and tarragon leaves.

2 Heat the oil in a large frying pan (skillet) and put in the spring onions (scallions). Cook for 1 minute, add the chops or fillets and cook for 2–3 minutes; turn over and cook for the same time on the other side.

3 Add the pears with the wine, vinegar and tarragon, together with a little seasoning. Continue cooking until the meat and pears are tender, then serve topped with the nuts and mint leaves. Rice noodles and Chinese cabbage (bok choy) are excellent accompaniments.

Variation: veal chops could be served in the same way. When buying veal, look for organic meat.

Freezing: do not freeze the cooked dish, but defrosted, well-dried meat could be used.

liver with prunes and herbs SERVES 4

Liver is packed with nutrients needed by a healthy digestive system (read more about liver in Chapter 4). Choose calf's liver if possible as it has a more delicate flavour and tender texture than lamb's liver. This recipe is good for either.

Ingredients

METRIC (IMPERIAL)		AMERICAN
about 8	ready-to-eat dried prunes	about 8
1 tablespoon	sun-dried tomatoes, finely chopped	1 tablespoon
140ml (¼ pint)	chicken stock	⅔ cup
2 tablespoons	olive oil	2½ tablespoons
2	garlic cloves, chopped	2
455g (1lb)	liver, thinly chopped	1lb
to taste	sea salt and freshly ground black pepper	to taste
2 tablespoons	Madeira or port wine	2½ tablespoons
1 tablespoon	chopped rosemary	1 tablespoon
1 tablespoon	chopped parsley	1 tablespoon

Method

1 Remove any stones from the prunes, slice the fruit and put, with the sun-dried tomatoes, into the stock to soak for 10 minutes. Do this even if the sun-dried tomatoes have been in oil.

2 Heat the oil in a large frying pan (skillet), add the garlic and cook gently for 3 minutes. Put in the liver and cook for 1 minute if using calf's liver, or 2 minutes with lamb's liver. Turn over and cook for the same time on the other side.

3 Add the prunes, sun-dried tomatoes and stock to the pan. Season well and bring to simmering point. Cook for 2 minutes then add the wine and herbs. Heat for 1 minute and serve with cooked rice or pasta and green vegetables.

Variations:

- *Use ready-to-eat dried apricots instead of prunes and a slightly sweet sherry instead of Madeira or port wine.*
- *Use the same amount of whole stoned dates instead of prunes.*

Veal Escalopes: thin slices of veal, cut from the fillet, can be cooked in the same way as the liver. The meat is equally good with ready-to-eat dried prunes or apricots. Veal must be cooked very thoroughly, so check on the cooking time at stages 2 and 3.

Freezing: the cooked dish should not be frozen but defrosted, well-dried liver or veal could be used.

honey and ginger chicken SERVES 4–5

A topping of honey gives chicken portions an inviting colour and helps keep the flesh moist. Finely grated ginger is suggested in the recipe but you could use ground ginger instead (see 'Variations').

Ingredients

METRIC (IMPERIAL)		AMERICAN
4	chicken breasts	4
2 tablespoons	olive oil	2½ tablespoons
2 tablespoons	thin honey	2½ tablespoons
5 level teaspoons or to taste	grated root ginger	5 level teaspoons or to taste
to taste	sea salt	to taste
	To garnish	
	watercress	

Method

1 Preheat the oven to 190°C/375°F/Gas Mark 5 or 170–180°C with a fan oven.

2 If you want to make the chicken easier to eat, cut out the breast bone then form the flesh back into an attractive shape. The skins can be left on the chicken or removed.

3 Brush the chicken with olive oil; mix the honey, ginger and a little salt then spread over the top of the breasts. Place in an ovenproof baking dish.

4 Bake uncovered for approximately 25 minutes or until the chicken is tender. Garnish with watercress; serve hot with Watercress Sauce (*see page 151*) and mixed vegetables. Top the chicken with any honey liquid left in the dish.

Variations:

- *If serving the chicken cold, mix some of the honey liquid with live yoghurt and chopped watercress leaves and use this as a dressing.*
- *Use 1 level teaspoon ground ginger instead of the grated root ginger. This topping can be put on a whole chicken but is better added during cooking so it does not burn. Roast the chicken for just over half the total cooking time and remove from the oven. Pour away any surplus fat then top the chicken breast with the honey and ginger and complete the roasting.*
- *Use grated horseradish or horseradish cream instead of ginger.*

Freezing: do not freeze the cooked dish. Frozen chicken could be used, but defrost and dry the portions well before adding the oil and honey coating.

chicken pockets SERVES 4–5

Chicken is an ideal food for people who are not feeling well but it can be boring if served too often. Add interest by cutting pockets into chicken portions and filling with a tasty stuffing; this also helps to keep the flesh moist. If you do not have time to make a stuffing, simply insert your favourite chopped herbs and thin slivers of lemon or orange zest plus a little olive oil or melted butter.

Good-sized chicken breasts are ideal; if you prefer darker meat, use the thighs. In either case the bones must be removed to make space for the filling. You can leave the skins on the joints as long as the person you are cooking for is able to deal with them.

Ingredients

METRIC (IMPERIAL)		AMERICAN
4	good-sized chicken portions	4
	stuffing as suggestions below	
1½ tablespoons	olive oil	scant 2 tablespoons
to taste	sea salt and freshly ground black pepper	to taste
	To garnish	
	mint or herb used in the stuffing	

SUGGESTED STUFFINGS:

Cheese and Mint: mint is a very important herb for a healthy gut so be generous with the amount you use. There are several different kinds of mint. My favourite is peppermint.

Blend 115–140g (4–5oz/½–⅝ cup) cream or curd cheese with 2 (2½) tablespoons chopped mint, 2 teaspoons lemon juice and a little seasoning.

You could use the same weight of grated cheese, softened with 1 tablespoon live yoghurt.

Rice, Chive and Pine Nut: blend 55g (2oz/good ⅓ cup) cooked and well-drained long-grain white rice with 1 tablespoon olive oil, 2 (2½) tablespoons finely snipped chives, 85g (3oz/¾cup) coarsely chopped pine nuts and seasoning to taste.

Ground Almond and Ginger: blend 55g (2oz/½ cup) ground almonds with 2–3 teaspoons grated root ginger, 1–2 teaspoons lemon or lime zest and 1 tablespoon lemon or lime juice. Add 1 tablespoon chopped basil and seasoning.

Method

1 Preheat the oven to 190°C/375°F/Gas Mark 5 or 170–180°C with a fan oven.

2 Remove the bones from each chicken portion, fill with the selected stuffing then form the flesh into a neat shape. You can insert a small wooden skewer or cocktail stick (toothpick) to ensure the joints do not open out in cooking.

3 Put into an ovenproof dish and add the oil, making sure this covers all parts of the chicken. Season to taste and cover the dish.

4 Bake for approximately 30 minutes or until the chicken is tender and the stuffing piping hot. Garnish with your chosen herb and serve hot or cold. If serving hot, have a selection of seasonal vegetables. If serving cold, choose a refreshing salad (*see pages 99 and 140*).

Variations:

- *Use boned quail or portions of pheasant or other game birds instead of chicken portions.*
- *Duck breasts could be filled in the same way, but always remove the skins. Fill with 'Rice, Chive and Pine Nut or Ground Almond and Ginger stuffings. Cheese makes an over-rich filling.*

Freezing: do not freeze the cooked dish. Defrosted frozen birds can be used.

cooking duck

Duck, or young duckling, makes a pleasant change from chicken. Although modern rearing methods produce birds that are leaner than in the past, they still have a high fat content. If you cook the bird correctly, and remove the skin before serving, you reduce the fat to a large extent. Many people like a crisp, brown skin on their duck, so whether to remove it is a matter of personal taste, or medical advice if on a low-fat diet.

Duck portions make it easier to serve the bird, as carving or jointing a whole duck is not the easiest of tasks.

Practically every fruit blends well with duck. The traditional apple or orange sauces are ideal but do try the less well-known blackcurrant sauce, given overleaf. The rich flavour of these berries blends wonderfully with duck.

duck with blackcurrant sauce SERVES 4

Ingredients

METRIC (IMPERIAL)		AMERICAN
4	duck breast portions	4
	Blackcurrant sauce	
225g (8oz)	blackcurrants	½lb
285ml (½ pint)	chicken stock, but see 'Variations'	1¼ cups
1 tablespoon	duck fat, see stage 2	1 tablespoon
2 tablespoons	clear honey	2½ tablespoons
1 tablespoon	redcurrant jelly (optional)	1 tablespoon
2 teaspoons	cornflour (cornstarch), or arrowroot	2 teaspoons
140ml (¼ pint)	water, but see stage 5	⅔ cup
to taste	sea salt and freshly ground black pepper	to taste

Method

1 Preheat the oven to 200°C/400°F/Gas Mark 6 or 180–190°C with a fan oven. Stand the duck portions on a rack, placed in a roasting tin.

2 Put the duck into the oven and cook for 15 minutes. Remove and prick the skin lightly with a fine skewer or fork. Do not prick deeply or the fat will soak inwards

instead of spurting out. You should be able to spoon out the tablespoon of fat from the tin to make the sauce. Replace the duck in the oven and continue cooking. You should prick again after another 10 minutes. The total cooking time will be about 40 minutes but check carefully as the duck should be thoroughly cooked. The skin will become brown and crisp.

3   **For the sauce**: start to make this the moment the duck portions are placed in the oven. Wash the blackcurrants in cold water, put into a saucepan with the stock. Simmer very gently until the berries are tender but unbroken.

4   Add the duck fat and honey – never sweeten blackcurrants until they are tender as the skins do not soften further when honey (or sugar) is added.

5   Stir in the redcurrant jelly if using and the cornflour or arrowroot blended with the water. Continue stirring over a low heat until the sauce thickens and becomes clear. Season very lightly. (For a puréed sauce, liquidize the ingredients, then reheat.)

6   Serve the duck with the sauce, new potatoes and peas plus crisp green salad leaves with slices of fresh orange.

Variations:

*   *If roasting a whole duck and you have the giblets, simmer these to provide duck stock and use instead of chicken stock.*

*   *If you do not want such a savoury sauce, use butter instead of duck fat and water instead of stock. Omit the seasoning.*

*   *To roast whole ducks, allow 15 minutes per 455g (1lb) plus an extra 15 minutes. Start cooking at the temperature in stage 1 but reduce to 190°C/375°F/Gas Mark 5 or 170–180°C with a fan oven after 1 hour. Prick the skin every 15 minutes.*

Freezing: do not freeze the cooked dish. Defrosted frozen duck could be used. The puréed version of the sauce freezes well.

tajine of quail SERVES 4–6

Quail is a small game bird that lends itself to this Arab recipe. The word tajine *is used to describe the special cooking dish with a pyramid-shaped lid used in Morocco, but you can use a saucepan or a covered casserole in the oven. The same word is used for the food served in the tajine. Try to buy boned quail, which is much easier to deal with than the whole birds.*

Ingredients

METRIC (IMPERIAL)		AMERICAN
8	boned quail	8
I teaspoon	ground cinnamon	I teaspoon
½ teaspoon	saffron powder	½ teaspoon
½ teaspoon	grated or ground nutmeg	½ teaspoon
I teaspoon	ground ginger	I teaspoon
2 tablespoons	olive oil	2½ tablespoons
455g (Ilb)	very small pickling onions	Ilb
570ml (1 pint)	water	2½ cups
2 tablespoons	clear honey	2½ tablespoons
few strips	orange zest	few strips
3 tablespoons	orange juice	3¾ tablespoons
to taste	sea salt and freshly ground black pepper	to taste
about 12	dates, stoned	about 12
85g (3oz)	whole almonds, blanched	good ½ cup

Method

1 Cut each quail into about 4 portions. Put all the spices into a dry, heavy saucepan and place over a very low heat for 3 minutes. Stir once or twice so they do not scorch.

2 Add the oil and mix with the spices. Heat then put in the onions and turn in the hot oil for about 5 minutes. Add the pieces of quail and turn around so they become coated with spiced oil. Pour in the water then add the honey, orange zest, juice and seasoning. Cover the pan tightly and simmer gently for 40 minutes.

3 Add the dates and nuts and cook for another 10 minutes or until the quail is very tender. Serve with couscous or rice and a green salad.

Variations:

- *To cook in the oven: preheat the oven to 170°C/325°F/Gas Mark 3 or 140–150°C with a fan oven. Follow stages 1 and 2. When the ingredients have been added, including seasoning, transfer to a casserole. Cover and cook for 45 minutes. Add the dates and nuts and cook for a further 10 minutes.*
- *Use diced guinea fowl – not a game bird but with a stronger taste than chicken – instead of quail or use diced pheasant.*
- *Use diced chicken instead of quail.*

Freezing: when cold, transfer to a freezer container. This tajine freezes well.

adding interest to vegetables

 Vegetables are an important part of any diet, and particularly so for a healthy gut. Here are a few ideas for adding interest to some of the vegetables recommended for the diet.

cabbages and greens

When cooking green vegetables, shred the leaves so they cook quickly and place them in the minimum of lightly salted boiling water, cooking for the shortest time possible so they retain flavour and texture. Tender leaves are excellent in salads.

With onion and apple: cut 1 or 2 small onions into thin slices and separate into rings. Peel, core and thinly slice 1 or 2 dessert apples. Cook both in a little olive oil. When the greens are cooked, drain and blend with the onion and apple mixture.

With caraway seeds: drain the cooked greens and mix with a little olive oil and 1 or 2 teaspoons caraway seeds.

With herbs: mix lightly cooked green vegetables with freshly chopped mint and parsley. These herbs are particularly good with Chinese cabbage (bok choy). This is a useful vegetable as it keeps well and is equally good cooked or raw in a salad.

With spices: flavour the water in which the greens are cooked with a little ground ginger or cinnamon. When cooked, top with live yoghurt and a sprinkling of the spices.

cauliflower and broccoli

With nuts: choose a contrasting colour for eye-appeal. Top green broccoli with blanched flaked almonds and white cauliflower with chopped walnuts.

Polonaise: this classic garnish is both health-giving and attractive. Top the cooked vegetables with chopped hard-boiled egg, chopped parsley and crisply fried breadcrumbs.

carrots

With orange: add shreds of orange zest to the cooking water or sprinkle finely grated orange zest over the vegetables in a steamer.

Gingered Carrots: add a little ground ginger to the cooking water or sprinkle the vegetables with finely chopped preserved ginger if cooked in a steamer.

Freezing: do not freeze. Defrosted uncooked vegetables can be used.

spiced coleslaw SERVES 4

Coleslaw is one of the most appetizing ways of serving cabbage. In the following version, important spices are added to make it particularly suitable as well as more interesting.

Ingredients

METRIC (IMPERIAL)		AMERICAN
	Spiced dressing	
3 tablespoons	Mayonnaise (see *page 157*)	3¾ tablespoons
½–1 teaspoon	ground ginger	½–1 teaspoon
¼ teaspoon	ground cinnamon	¼ teaspoon
pinch	cayenne pepper	pinch
1 tablespoon	extra virgin olive oil	1 tablespoon
1 tablespoon	lemon juice	1 tablespoon
to taste	sea salt and freshly ground black pepper	to taste
	Salad	
¼–½	white cabbage or firm cabbage heart	¼–½
1	large dessert apple	1
2	medium carrots	2
2 tablespoons	chopped spring onions (scallions)	2½ tablespoons
2 tablespoons	chopped parsley	2½ tablespoons

Method

1 Mix all the dressing ingredients together. Put into a bowl.
2 Finely shred the cabbage by hand or with a shredding attachment on a food processor or electric mixer.
3 Core but do not peel the apple, wash it well in cold water and dry it. Cut into neat, small dice and put into the dressing, so the fruit does not discolour.
4 Grate the carrots and add to the dressing with the spring onions (scallions) and parsley. Lastly mix in the cabbage, stirring well to make sure all the ingredients are well moistened. Spoon into the salad bowl.

Variations:

- *Use all live yoghurt instead of Mayonnaise or use half yoghurt and half Mayonnaise.*
- *Add about 55g (2oz/½ cup) coarsely chopped walnuts or pecan or pine nuts.*
- *Add about 4 (5) tablespoons finely chopped celery.*
- *Add several slices of pineapple (finely diced) instead of the apple or use both apple and pineapple.*
- ***Herb Dressing****: add 2 (2½) tablespoons chopped mint and 1 tablespoon chopped parsley to the dressing and omit the ginger and cinnamon.*

Freezing: not recommended.

roast garlic SERVES 4

Garlic is a healing vegetable known to fight infection and lower blood cholesterol levels. Some people dislike its strong flavour, and this is when roasted garlic can be served. By roasting the garlic in the oven it acquires a wonderfully mellow taste and an almost buttery consistency. When recipes list fresh garlic, you could omit this and add some roasted garlic to the other ingredients when they are softened. The soft garlic makes a delicious accompaniment to many savoury dishes; simply arrange a spoonful on top of cooked poultry or other foods.

Ingredients

METRIC (IMPERIAL)		AMERICAN
2	large garlic heads	2
2 tablespoons	olive oil	2½ tablespoons

Method

1 Preheat the oven to 190°C/375°F/Gas Mark 5 or 170–180°C with a fan oven.

2 Pull away the garlic cloves from each head. I like to remove the skins from each clove but many people roast the garlic with the skin on, and it does become quite soft when cooked. If you do not like the skins, it is easier to remove them before cooking.

3 Pour the oil into an ovenproof dish or tin and heat for about 5 minutes in the oven. Add the garlic and turn in the oil until each clove is well coated. Roast for 20–25 minutes or until as soft as required. The garlic turns a pleasing golden colour.

Freezing: not recommended.

lime and mint lentil loaf SERVES 4–6

Lentils make a good vegetarian dish, and the lime and mint enhance their health value. There is no need to buy the expensive Puy lentils for this loaf but, if you are planning to have a lentil salad, then Puy lentils are the ones to choose. Cook them until only just firm, cool and serve with mixed salad ingredients. This loaf is excellent hot or cold.

Ingredients

METRIC (IMPERIAL)		AMERICAN
2 tablespoons	olive or sunflower oil	2½ tablespoons
2	medium onions, finely chopped	2
2	medium dessert apples, peeled, cored and finely chopped	2
550ml (18fl oz)	water	2¼ cups
1 level tablespoon	finely grated lime zest	1 level tablespoon
3 tablespoons	lime juice	3¾ tablespoons
225g (8oz)	split lentils	1 cup
to taste	salt and freshly ground black pepper	to taste
3 tablespoons	finely chopped mint	3¾ tablespoons
½ teaspoon	ground cumin	½ teaspoon
55g (2oz)	rolled oats	scant ⅔ cup
55g (2oz)	raisins	⅓ cup
50 g (2 oz)	chopped walnuts, optional	½ cup
1	large egg, whisked	1

Method

1 Heat the oil in a saucepan, add the onions and cook gently for 5 minutes, then add the apples and turn in the fat.

2 Pour in the water with the lime zest and juice and bring to the boil. Add the lentils and mix well with the other ingredients. Season and cover the pan. Simmer steadily for 30 minutes or until the lentils are almost tender and the liquid has been absorbed. If any liquid is left, strain the ingredients but make sure they are moist.

3 Stir in the remaining ingredients, taste and add extra seasoning if required. Mix very thoroughly then spoon into a greased 900g (2lb) loaf tin or oval casserole. Preheat the oven to 180°C/350°F/Gas Mark 4 or 160–170°C with a fan oven.

4   Do not cover the tin or casserole. Bake for 45 minutes or until the loaf is golden
    brown and firm on the top. Cool in the baking container for 5 minutes, then turn
    out. Serve hot with seasonal vegetables and Lime Mint Sauce (*see page 154*) or cold
    with salad and Mayonnaise (*see page 157*); this can be flavoured with chopped mint.

Variations: instead of using rolled oats, add the same weight (or 2 cups) of soft
breadcrumbs.

Ginger Lentil Loaf: use 570ml (1 pint/2½ cups) water and omit both lime zest and
juice. The chopped mint can be retained or replaced by chopped parsley. Add 1
teaspoon ground ginger at stage 3 with 4 (5) tablespoons diced preserved ginger. The
raisins and nuts can be retained.

Sesame Lentil Loaf: use 1 tablespoon olive oil and 1 tablespoon sesame seed oil at
stage 1. Omit the lime zest and juice and use 570ml (1 pint/2½ cups) water. Replace the
chopped mint with chopped parsley and add 1 tablespoon sesame seeds at stage 3. The
raisins can be replaced by chopped dates, and the walnuts with chopped pine nuts.

Freezing: the first loaf and any of the variations freeze well. If you are catering for a
small family it may be a good idea to mark the loaf into portions and separate these with
baking parchment, so one portion may be removed without defrosting the whole loaf.

savoury accompaniments

 These savoury sauces, salsas and dressings are an excellent way of incorporating some important health-giving ingredients into a meal. Recipes for sweet accompaniments begin on page 202.

onion marmalade

'Marmalade' may seem a strange term for an onion mixture, but the onions are cut in a similar way to the peel of oranges or other citrus fruit for the popular preserve. This savoury-sweet mixture is excellent with fish, meat, poultry and game. When making the marmalade for the first time, it may be wise to choose a mild-flavoured onion. You can change this on subsequent occasions if you desire a stronger taste. All members of the onion family should be included in your diet whenever possible.

Ingredients

METRIC (IMPERIAL)		AMERICAN
1 tablespoon	olive oil	1 tablespoon
55g (2oz)	butter	¼ cup
680g (1½lb)	onions, peeled and thinly sliced, NOT chopped	1½lb
½ teaspoon	sea salt	½ teaspoon
generous shake	freshly ground black pepper	generous shake
1 teaspoon	finely grated lemon zest	1 teaspoon
1 teaspoon	chopped rosemary	1 teaspoon
1 teaspoon	chopped basil	1 teaspoon
1 fresh	bay leaf	1 fresh
½–1 teaspoon	ground cinnamon	½–1 teaspoon
115g (4oz)	soft brown sugar	scant ½ cup
2 tablespoons	red wine vinegar	2½ tablespoons
1 tablespoon	balsamic vinegar	1 tablespoon
2 tablespoons	sweet sherry	2½ tablespoons

Method

1 Heat the olive oil and butter in a saucepan, taking care that they do not become too hot. Add the onions and stir well until coated with the oil and butter.

2 Add seasoning, zest, herbs and spice. Stir over a low heat for 5 minutes then cover the saucepan; allow to cook slowly for 25 minutes. Check from time to time to make sure the mixture is not sticking to the pan.

3 Stir in the sugar and continue stirring until dissolved. Add the rest of the ingredients and continue simmering in the uncovered pan until they form a thick mixture.

4   Spoon into heated jars or containers, cover and store for up to 2½ weeks in the refrigerator.

Freezing: this mixture freezes well. Allow an air space of about 2cm (¾ inch) in the containers as the liquid content makes the mixture expand as it freezes.

Variations:

- *For a hot flavour add 1 or 2 (2½) tablespoons finely chopped red chillies at stage 1.*
- *For a sweeter flavour add 85g (3oz/½ cup) chopped dates or raisins at stage 1.*
- *Use half sugar and half clear honey.*

salsas

The term 'salsa' is often taken to mean a sauce, but that is not quite true. A salsa is not a pouring sauce but a mixture of ingredients to accompany main dishes. Although the texture is pleasantly moist, it is not of a consistency to pour over food. Generally the ingredients are uncooked and retain their firm texture. Fruit, vegetables and spices are included in the interesting mixtures. You will have no difficulty in creating your own appetizing salsas if you refer to the list of recommended foods on pages 54–5. Here are several recipes that combine interesting and health-giving ingredients. Serve salsas in small dishes. Do not freeze any of the following salsa mixtures.

beetroot (beet) and apple salsa SERVES 4

This is particularly good with wild or ordinary duck or with game birds.

Ingredients

METRIC (IMPERIAL)		AMERICAN
225g (8oz)	cooked beetroot, skinned	½lb
2	large dessert apples, peeled and cored	2
4	celery sticks	4
3 tablespoons	chopped spring onions (scallions)	scant 4 tablespoons
2 tablespoons	finely chopped mint	2½ tablespoons
I tablespoon	lime or lemon juice	I tablespoon
2 tablespoons	extra virgin olive oil	2½ tablespoons
2 teaspoons	balsamic or sherry vinegar	2 teaspoons
to taste	sea salt and freshly ground black pepper	to taste

Method

1 Cut the beetroot, apples and celery into 1.5–2cm (½–¾ inch) dice and mix with all the other ingredients.

Variations:

- *The above ingredients make an excellent salad if placed on a base of watercress, rocket and lettuce leaves.*
- *Add a good pinch of chilli powder or 1–2 teaspoons finely chopped red chilli.*

buckwheat and fruit salsa SERVES 4–5

Buckwheat (kasha) is not a wheat but a member of the rhubarb family. It gives a wonderfully satisfying texture to this salsa, which is excellent with most meats or fish.

Ingredients

METRIC (IMPERIAL)		AMERICAN
115g (4oz)	buckwheat, as coarse as possible	½ cup
285ml (½ pint)	water	1⅓ cups
½ teaspoon	ground cinnamon, see stage 3	½ teaspoon
2	large, ripe but firm bananas	2
2	large, ripe but firm pears	2
2 tablespoons	lime or lemon juice	2½ tablespoons
4 tablespoons	grapes, halved and de-seeded if necessary	5 tablespoons
3 tablespoons	pine nuts, coarsely chopped	scant 4 tablespoons
2 tablespoons	finely chopped basil	2½ tablespoons
3 tablespoons	live yoghurt	scant 4 tablespoons
2 teaspoons	grated horseradish	2 teaspoons

Method

1 Place the buckwheat in a bowl. Bring the water to the boil, pour over the buckwheat, add the cinnamon and stir to blend. Leave until the buckwheat is quite cold, then strain and discard any moisture. Place the buckwheat on a flat dish and leave until dry.

2 Peel the bananas, cut into 3.5cm (1½ inch) slices and quarter each slice. Peel and core the pears, and cut into 1.5cm (½ inch) dice. Mix the two fruits with the lime or lemon juice then add the rest of the ingredients, including the cold buckwheat.

3 Taste the mixture and add more ground cinnamon if desired.

Variations:

• *Use horseradish cream if horseradish is not available.*
• *Use diced kiwi fruit instead of grapes.*

spiced vegetable salsa SERVES 4–6

The ginger gives this mixture a really piquant, hot taste.

Ingredients

METRIC (IMPERIAL)		AMERICAN
¼–½	small cauliflower	¼–½
to taste	sea salt and freshly ground black pepper	to taste
3 tablespoons	virgin olive oil	scant 4 tablespoons
2 tablespoons	grated root ginger	2½ tablespoons
about 12	small spring onions (scallions)	about 12
6 tablespoons	chopped celery from the heart	7½ tablespoons
3	medium carrots, coarsely grated	3
1 tablespoon	balsamic vinegar	1 tablespoon
2 teaspoons	clear honey	2 teaspoons
2 tablespoons	chopped parsley	2½ tablespoons

Method

1 Remove about 12 very small florets from the cauliflower. Put into well-seasoned boiling water and cook for 2 minutes only, then drain. While hot, place in the olive oil in a large bowl. Leave until cold.

2 Add the rest of the ingredients. If the spring onions (scallions) are very small they can be left whole, just remove all the green stems. If slightly larger, they can be halved.

Variations:

- *Use half chopped preserved ginger and half grated root ginger.*
- *This makes an excellent vegetable salad if placed on a bed of rocket or dandelion leaves, which are extremely valuable on this diet. The vegetable mixture can be made more moist by adding a little live yoghurt or crème fraîche. You can top the salad with a sprinkling of caraway seeds.*

savoury sauces

In the past most sauces were based on a butter and flour roux, with the addition of milk and cream or other liquids. Today's sauces tend to be lighter and full of interesting flavours, such as Pesto (*see page 155*). However, there may be times when you need to take more milk. The Hot Watercress Sauce and the other herb sauces that follow are good examples of dairy-based sauces with plenty of flavour that are not unduly thick.

hot watercress sauce SERVES 4

Watercress is a wonderfully healthy ingredient with an interesting flavour. Read more about this, and the value of other herbs, in Chapter 4. The stalks provide most of the flavour, so they should not be discarded but used in stage 1. If you want to reduce the fat content, use skimmed milk. You will see I have suggested a little less flour than in standard recipes to give a more modern consistency.

Ingredients

METRIC (IMPERIAL)		AMERICAN
I good-sized bunch	watercress	I good-sized bunch
285ml (½ pint) plus extra	milk	1⅓ cups plus extra
30g (Ioz)	butter or margarine	2 tablespoons
20g (¾oz)	plain (all-purpose) flour	scant ¼ cup
to taste	sea salt and freshly ground black pepper	to taste
I tablespoon or to taste	lemon juice	I tablespoon or to taste

Method

1   Wash the watercress in cold water and dry well. Cut off the stalks, place in the milk and bring to boiling point. Remove from the heat and allow to stand for about 30 minutes. Strain into a measuring jug and add enough milk to make 285ml (½ pint/1⅓ cups) again. Discard the stalks, which will have imparted a slightly mustard flavour to the milk.

2 Chop the watercress leaves. Heat the butter or margarine in a saucepan, stir in the flour, then add the milk. Whisk or stir briskly as the sauce comes to the boil and thickens. Allow to simmer gently for 2 or 3 minutes, then add the watercress leaves and seasoning to taste. Make sure the sauce is very hot but do not cook for any length of time. Check the consistency; if too thick, add a little more milk. Remove from the heat and whisk in the lemon juice.

This sauce is excellent with fish, poultry and an omelette.

Variations:
- *Use half milk and half stock – the stock should be compatible with the main dish, e.g. chicken stock with poultry.*
- *If you do not eat wheat then use cornflour (cornstarch) or potato flour (fecule) to thicken the sauce instead of flour. Use half the quantity of cornflour, as it has better thickening qualities than flour; use the same amount of potato flour as for wheat flour.*
- *A small amount of double (heavy) cream could be added to the hot or cold sauce.*

Cold Watercress Sauce: Mix chopped watercress leaves with live yoghurt, season well and add a sprinkling of lemon or lime juice. A little Dijon mustard emphasizes the mustard flavour.

This is excellent with hot or cold fish dishes.

Variations: herbs of various kinds can be used instead of watercress in the hot or cold sauces above. Here are some of the most interesting.

Parsley Sauce: this sauce was widely used in the past, so much so that it fell out of favour. However, parsley gives an excellent flavour, particularly if you choose the flat-leaved variety. As you will see in Chapter 4, parsley is packed with minerals and vitamins that strengthen the digestive system. Follow the recipes for the watercress sauces above but use about 3 (3¾) tablespoons chopped parsley instead of watercress. The stalks could be infused in the milk as in Hot Watercress Sauce. The lemon juice can be omitted.

Fennel Sauce: omit the watercress and add 3 (3¾) tablespoons chopped fennel leaves in either the Hot or Cold Watercress Sauce. To make a more interesting texture, also add 2 (2½) tablespoons finely chopped and grated raw fennel root. The lemon juice blends well with fennel. This sauce is particularly good with fish.

Creamy Mint Sauce: this version of mint sauce makes a pleasant change. Use approximately 2 (2½) tablespoons chopped mint leaves instead of watercress in the hot or cold sauces above. The stalks of the mint can be infused in the milk. Add the lemon juice as given in Hot Watercress Sauce and serve with lamb, poultry or fish. The recipe overleaf provides another unusual Mint Sauce.

Sorrel Sauce: a less well-known herb than many, sorrel looks like spinach but has a more bitter taste. To make the sauce cook about 115g (4oz/¼lb) young sorrel leaves in boiling, salted water for 4 minutes. Strain and discard the liquid. Sieve or liquidize (blend) the sorrel leaves then add them gradually to the hot basic sauce instead of the watercress. The lemon juice is not necessary. Do not add too much sorrel without checking the flavour as it is very much an acquired taste. This sauce is a perfect accompaniment to cooked fish.

Adding more flavour: a little ground ginger, ground cinnamon or grated nutmeg can be added to any of the sauces above.

Freezing: not recommended.

lime mint sauce SERVES 4

This sauce blends well with the Lentil Loaf on page 143 and makes an interesting change from ordinary mint sauce.

Ingredients

METRIC (IMPERIAL)		AMERICAN
2 teaspoons	finely grated lemon zest	2 teaspoons
2 tablespoons	boiling water	2½ tablespoons
2 tablespoons	caster sugar	2½ tablespoons
6 tablespoons	finely chopped mint leaves	7½ tablespoons
3 tablespoons	lime juice	3¾ tablespoons
5 tablespoons or to taste	white wine vinegar	6¼ tablespoons or to taste

Method

Put the lemon zest into a basin, add the boiling water and sugar and leave until cold, then add the remaining ingredients.

Variations:
- *Use lemon zest and juice instead of lime.*
- *Use rice vinegar instead of white wine vinegar.*

Freezing: this freezes well although the mint does lose some taste and texture.

pesto SERVES 4–8

Pesto has become one of today's favourite sauces. It can be served with a great variety of foods, such as cooked pasta, vegetables, egg dishes, salads and soups. It is an uncooked sauce, assembled in a liquidizer (blender) or food processor. The classic ingredients are given in the following recipe. Home-made Pesto is completely different from the many commercial versions available. Its flavour is fresh and delicious. Basil is one of the important herbs for a healthy gut, but if you find its flavour slightly too strong, mix parsley leaves and/or mint and marjoram leaves with a smaller amount of basil (see also 'Variations'). The number of servings will vary according to the size of the main food.

Ingredients

METRIC (IMPERIAL)		AMERICAN
about 36	small basil leaves	about 36
I or 2	garlic cloves	I or 2
85g (3oz)	Parmesan cheese, grated	I cup
55g (2oz)	Pecorino cheese, grated	¼ cup
6 tablespoons	extra virgin olive oil	7½ tablespoons
100g (3½oz)	pine nuts	good ¾ cup
to taste	salt and freshly ground black pepper	to taste

Method

1 Tear the leaves into slightly smaller pieces and put into the liquidizer (blender) or food processor with the garlic. Switch on for a few seconds.

2 Put in the cheeses and once again process for a few seconds.

3 Leave the motor running and gradually add the oil, which will begin to thicken the sauce. Add the nuts and a little seasoning.

Variations:

- *As mentioned at the top of the page, other herbs can be used.*
- *If serving with fish, use some fennel or dill leaves and a small piece of finely chopped fennel root.*
- *Substitute almonds or other nuts for pine nuts.*
- *You can make a richer sauce by adding up to 55g (2oz/¼ cup) of melted butter at the end of stage 2.*
- *Pecorino cheese can be omitted or a mild Cheddar substituted.*

Freezing: not recommended.

aiöli SERVES 6

This French garlic dressing is a classic topping for fish soups but is also an excellent alternative to Mayonnaise.

Ingredients

METRIC (IMPERIAL)		AMERICAN
4	large garlic cloves	4
2	egg yolks, from large eggs	2
to taste	sea salt and freshly ground black pepper	to taste
up to 230ml (8fl oz)	extra virgin olive oil	up to I cup
I tablespoon	lemon juice or white wine or rice vinegar	I tablespoon
I tablespoon	boiling water, optional	I tablespoon

Method

1 Peel and crush the garlic cloves. The best way to crush them by hand is to place them in a mortar (heavy bowl) and crush them with a pestle. Another way is to sprinkle a little salt onto a chopping board (this helps to keep the garlic in place) and crush each clove separately with a heavy-bladed knife. Place the crushed garlic in an ordinary bowl.

2 Blend in the first egg yolk then the second and season well. Add the oil drop by drop (*see under Mayonnaise, opposite page*) then stir in the lemon juice or vinegar and boiling water. Store in a tightly covered container in the refrigerator for 2–3 days.

Freezing: not recommended.

mayonnaise SERVES 4–6

If you make your own Mayonnaise you can incorporate valuable foods into the dressing and ensure there are no preservatives. This recipe contains a good amount of olive oil, which is well known for its healthy properties. However, as you will be using uncooked eggs, it is important to ensure there is no reason to avoid them. If worried, make the Hard-boiled (Hard-cooked) Egg Mayonnaise (given overleaf) or the Tofu Mayonnaise on page 159. Choose organic olive oil if possible. To reduce the amount of fat, use light olive oil.

Ingredients

METRIC (IMPERIAL)		AMERICAN
2	egg yolks, from large eggs	2
1 teaspoon	Dijon mustard or English mustard (powder mixed with water or used from a tube)	1 teaspoon
to taste	sea salt and freshly ground black pepper	to taste
up to 285ml (½ pint)	extra virgin olive oil	up to 1⅓ cups
3 teaspoons	lemon juice or vinegar*	3 teaspoons
1 tablespoon	very hot water, optional	1 tablespoon

*White wine vinegar or rice vinegar are both excellent.

Method

1   Make quite sure the bowl in which you mix the dressing is absolutely dry. Add the egg yolks, mustard and seasoning; stir briskly.

2   Gradually incorporate the oil, drop by drop, beating well as you do so. If by chance the mixture shows signs of curdling (separating), stop adding the oil at once. Whisk briskly and the mixture should become smooth once again. If it does not, break a third egg yolk into another bowl and add the curdled mixture drop by drop. It will then become thick and smooth again. The more oil you add, the thicker the dressing becomes.

3   When sufficient oil for your taste has been used, stir in the lemon juice or vinegar. The water is not essential but it makes a more delicate dressing. This should be stirred briskly into the other ingredients. Taste and adjust the seasoning. Use at once or cover and store in the refrigerator for 2–3 days.

Variations:

Hard-boiled (Hard-cooked) Egg Mayonnaise: hard-boil 2 eggs and use the yolks instead of the raw yolks in the recipe above. Continue just as the method given. For a creamier texture, first blend the hard-boiled egg yolks with 2 tablespoons single (light) cream, then add the mustard, seasoning, olive oil and other ingredients, as above.

Liquidizer Mayonnaise: when making the Mayonnaise this way you can use 2 whole uncooked eggs rather than just the yolks or you can use the hard-boiled yolks (not the whites). Put the eggs or yolks into the goblet or food processor and add the mustard and seasoning. With the motor running on a low speed, gradually trickle the oil through the hole in the lid or funnel. You cannot use quite as much oil when incorporating whole eggs, rather than just the yolks. Lastly add the lemon juice or vinegar and hot water if required.

Freezing: not recommended.

tofu mayonnaise SERVES 4

Tofu (bean curd) is produced from soya beans and makes a first-class form of vegetable protein. This dressing has an interesting flavour and is lower in fat than ordinary mayonnaise. If possible, use the silken (softer) type of tofu.

Ingredients

METRIC (IMPERIAL)		AMERICAN
200g (7oz)	tofu	I cup
I teaspoon	Dijon mustard	I teaspoon
to taste	salt and freshly ground black pepper	to taste
I tablespoon	lemon juice or wine or rice vinegar	I tablespoon
3–5 tablespoons	extra virgin olive oil	3¾ to 6½ tablespoons

Method

1 If using ordinary tofu, cut it into very small pieces. Silken tofu is not so difficult to make smooth so chopping it is less important. Put the tofu into a bowl with the mustard, seasoning, lemon juice or vinegar and pound until smooth. A mortar is ideal for this purpose.

2 Gradually beat in the olive oil, drop by drop, until the required consistency is achieved. Use within 2–3 days and store in the refrigerator in a covered container.

Variations:

- *Use a liquidizer (blender) or food processor. Put the tofu and the other ingredients, except the olive oil, into the goblet or bowl and process until evenly blended and smooth. With the motor running on a low speed, gradually trickle the oil through the hole in the lid or funnel.*

- *The suggestions overleaf for adding flavour to a Vinaigrette Dressing are also successful with Tofu Mayonnaise.*

Freezing: not recommended.

vinaigrette dressing SERVES 4–6

This dressing is a partner to many salads, and its flavour can make a great deal of difference to the appeal of a dish. The first recipe gives the classic dressing but this can be varied in a number of ways. Under 'Variations' you will find suggestions for incorporating interesting ingredients known to benefit various digestive ailments. More information about these can be found in Chapter 4.

If you decide to use vinegar rather than lemon juice (an important ingredient on the diet), try rice vinegar. This has an excellent taste and is less acidic than wine vinegars.

Ingredients

METRIC (IMPERIAL)		AMERICAN
I teaspoon	Dijon mustard	I teaspoon
140ml (¼ pint)	extra virgin or virgin olive oil	⅔ cup
4 tablespoons	lemon juice or wine or rice vinegar	5 tablespoons
to taste	sea salt and freshly ground black pepper	to taste
I teaspoon	honey or sugar	I teaspoon

Method

1 Put all the ingredients into a bowl and whisk together, or put into a screw-topped jar, cover and shake briskly. The ingredients can also be mixed in a liquidizer (blender) or food processor.

2 Use as required. This dressing keeps well in a covered container for several days in a cool place.

Variations:

Change proportions of oil and lemon juice or vinegar, according to personal taste and the flavour of the food with which the dressing is to be used. A salad or other dish served with rather rich food may taste better with a smaller amount of oil, giving a sharper taste.

Change vinegar: substitute up to 1 tablespoon balsamic vinegar for the same amount of lemon juice or wine vinegar. Sherry vinegar could be substituted in the same way. Some red or white wines can be used instead of all vinegars.

Change oil: if you find olive oil too heavy; use light olive oil or mix olive oil with sunflower oil. Use up to 1 tablespoon sesame seed oil instead of all olive oil, and add up to 1 tablespoon sesame seeds to the dressing. Use walnut oil or other nut oils; I like half these and half olive oil. You could add appropriate chopped nuts, such as walnuts, to the dressing.

Add herbs: stir 2–3 (2½–3¾) tablespoons crushed garlic, mint, basil or tarragon into the dressing. If using Roast Garlic (*see page 142*) then use about double this amount.

Add spices: ½–1 teaspoon ground ginger, galangal or cinnamon could be added. Instead of ground ginger add 1–2 teaspoons grated root ginger or 3 teaspoons chopped stem ginger for a slightly sweet taste.

Alter seasonings: whole-grain mustard and some other commercial mustards can be used. Change the black pepper to cayenne or paprika.

Freezing: not recommended.

yoghurt dressing SERVES 4

This makes a tasty accompaniment to salads or savoury dishes. When buying the live yoghurt, choose the thickest variety available as this will produce the right consistency. The dressing can be prepared in a liquidizer (blender) or food processor but it tends to become thinner in consistency than when mixed by hand.

Ingredients

METRIC (IMPERIAL)		AMERICAN
285ml (½ pint)	thick live yoghurt	1⅓ cups
1 teaspoon	Dijon mustard	1 teaspoon
to taste	sea salt and freshly ground black pepper	to taste
1 tablespoon or to taste	lemon juice or white wine or rice vinegar	1 tablespoon or to taste
1–2 teaspoons	honey or sugar	1–2 teaspoons
3–4 tablespoons	extra virgin olive oil	3¾–5 tablespoons

Method

Put all the ingredients, except the olive oil, into a bowl and mix thoroughly, then whisk in the olive oil, drop by drop. Use at once or store for just 1 day in the refrigerator.

Variations:

Add chopped mint, other herbs or the additional ingredients given under *Vinaigrette Dressing* (*see page 160*). You can add 2–3 (2½–3¾) tablespoons finely chopped mint. This herb blends very well with many sweet ingredients.

Sweet Yoghurt Dressing: omit the seasoning and lemon juice. The yoghurt can be given more flavour with a little sweet sherry or sweet white wine and sugar or honey to taste. Serve with fruit salad or other desserts.

Raita: a usual accompaniment to curries, raita is equally good with savoury meat, fish or vegetable dishes. If you can eat cucumber on your diet, blend 285ml (10floz/1⅓ cups) thick live yoghurt with 5–6 (6¼–7½) tablespoons peeled and grated or finely chopped cucumber and 3 (3¾) tablespoons chopped mint. Season to taste.

- *Instead of cucumber, substitute finely chopped, diced fennel root. A few chopped fennel leaves can be included as well as the chopped mint.*
- *Instead of mint, you could use a mixture of basil and parsley, both important herbs.*
- *You could replace the mint or the herbs mentioned above with 2 (2½) tablespoons chopped tarragon.*
- *If serving Raita with a mildly flavoured dish, you could add a little grated horseradish or horseradish cream to the other ingredients.*

Freezing: not recommended.

pasta and rice dishes

 Pasta is made from hard durum wheat. If you are intolerant to wheat or advised not to eat it, you can buy gluten-free pasta. Rice noodles are also available.

There is such a variety of pasta shapes and sauces that you will have no difficulty in making dishes based on the recommended foods (see pages 54–5).

Remember not to overcook either pasta or rice. They lose flavour as well as texture when over-soft.

penne w vegetables

*Always use sufficient ach 115g (4oz/¼lb) of pasta you need at least 1.2 litres (2 pints/5 *

Ingredients

METRIC (IMPERIAL)		AMERICAN
2.4 litres (4 pints)	water	10 cups
to taste	sea salt	to taste
225g (8oz)	penne or other pasta	½lb
	Stir-fry Vegetables	
2 tablespoons	olive oil	2½ tablespoons
2	red (bell) peppers, deseeded and cut into large portions	2
2	courgettes (zucchini), sliced	2
3	medium tomatoes, skinned and coarsely chopped*	3
about 12	asparagus spears, trimmed	about 12
2 tablespoons	white wine or water with a squeeze of lemon juice	2½ tablespoons
few drops	Tabasco sauce, optional	few drops
to taste	sea salt and freshly ground black pepper	to taste
	Topping	
	herbs	
	Parmesan cheese, thinly shredded	

* Choose plum tomatoes if possible.

Method

1 Bring the water to the boil, add 1–2 level teaspoons salt, or to taste, then add the pasta and cook as the timing on the packet or until *al dente* (firm to the bite).
2 **Stir-fry Vegetables:** start to prepare these in plenty of time so the cooked pasta is not kept waiting. Heat the oil in a wok or a large frying pan (skillet). Add the peppers and courgettes (zucchini) and stir-fry for 3 minutes. Put in the tomatoes

and cook for a further minute, then add the asparagus spears. These should have been trimmed until the inedible tough base of each spear has been removed.

3 Continue stir-frying until the vegetables are tender but retain plenty of texture. Mix the wine, or water and lemon juice, with the Tabasco sauce, add to the pan with seasoning and heat for 1 minute.

4 Strain the penne, mix with the vegetables and top with the herbs and cheese.

Variations:

- *Choose other vegetables in season.*
- *Omit the tomatoes and flavour the vegetables with some Pesto (see page 155).*
- *Use canned plum tomatoes instead of fresh.*
- *Use sliced globe artichoke hearts in place of asparagus.*

Freezing: not recommended.

lamb pilaf SERVES 4–6

A pilaf, also known as a pilau, is made with long-grain rice. In this dish, the rice separates rather than forming a creamy texture. Basmati rice is excellent for this recipe; always wash thoroughly in cold water before using. This dish is an excellent way of serving cooked meat in an interesting manner. Store cooked or uncooked meat in the refrigerator until ready to use; do not leave in the warmth of the kitchen. Meat, poultry and game should be chopped or diced on a special chopping board, not one that is used for general purposes.

Ingredients

METRIC (IMPERIAL)		AMERICAN
2	large onions, cut into rings	2
2 tablespoons	olive or sunflower oil	2½ tablespoons
225g (8oz)	long-grain rice	1⅛ cups
570ml (1 pint)	lamb or chicken stock	2½ cups
1 tablespoon	chopped mint	1 tablespoon
1 tablespoon	chopped parsley	1 tablespoon
to taste	sea salt and freshly ground black pepper	to taste
455g (1lb)	cooked lamb, neatly diced	1lb
55g (2oz)	pine nuts or blanched almonds	½ cup
85g (3oz)	raisins or chopped dates	½ cup
	To garnish	
2	eggs, hard-boiled and shelled	2
	chopped parsley	

Method

1 Cut the onion rings in halves or quarters but do not chop finely. Heat the oil in a large pan, add the onions and cook gently for 6–7 minutes, or until tender.

2 Add the rice and stir into the onions, making sure all the grains are coated with oil. Pour in all the stock, adding the mint and parsley together with a little seasoning. Cover the pan, simmer for 15 minutes, stir once or twice and check the liquid carefully as it will evaporate rapidly if the heat is too high.

3 At the end of this time the rice should be getting soft, so add the meat, nuts and raisins or dates. Continue cooking until the meat is very hot. This is most important: when reheating meat it is essential this is done thoroughly. Taste and

adjust with seasoning. Top with sliced eggs and parsley. Serve with a green vegetable or salad.

Variations:

Chicken Pilaf: use cooked chicken instead of lamb and flavour the pilaf with parsley and chopped rosemary leaves or tarragon. The chicken flesh should be neatly diced.

Beef Pilaf: use cooked beef instead of lamb and flavour the beef or chicken stock with 2 teaspoons grated horseradish and the chopped parsley. Omit the mint. If you have no fresh horseradish then use 1 tablespoon horseradish cream. If you do not like horseradish, use 1 teaspoon ground ginger instead. The seasoning can include a little English mustard powder mixed with water or used from a tube. While you can dice the beef, it tends to be better coarsely minced.

Freezing: not recommended.

vegetable and nut risotto SERVES 4

A good risotto should have a creamy texture. Use arborio rice, or another medium-grain rice, and add the liquid gradually, as outlined below. The nuts provide protein but other foods can be used instead (see 'Variations'). The selection of vegetables adds colour as well as flavour to the rice.

Ingredients

METRIC (IMPERIAL)		AMERICAN
750ml (1¼ pints)	vegetable stock or water	generous 3 cups
2 tablespoons	sun-dried tomatoes, chopped	2½ tablespoons
2 tablespoons	olive or sunflower oil	2½ tablespoons
2	medium onions, chopped	2
2	garlic cloves, chopped	2
2	small courgettes (zucchini), diced	2
2	medium carrots, diced	2
1	red (bell) pepper, deseeded and diced	1
2	small leeks, thinly sliced	2
170g (6oz)	arborio rice	generous ¾ cup
to taste	sea salt and freshly ground black pepper	to taste
4 tablespoons	shelled peas	5 tablespoons
2 tablespoons	chopped parsley	2½ tablespoons
115g (4oz)	walnuts, chopped	1 cup
30g (1oz)	butter	2 tablespoons

To garnish

chopped parsley

shredded or grated Parmesan cheese

Method

1 Pour the stock or water into a small saucepan. If the sun-dried tomatoes are dry-packed, add to the stock. If they are in olive oil, remove from the oil, chop and put on one side to add towards the end of the cooking time. When you start to make the risotto, the stock should be heated and kept warm until all of it is used.

2 Heat the oil in a good-sized saucepan. Add the onions and cook gently for 5 minutes, then add the garlic and all the other vegetables, except the peas if they are young. Heat the vegetables slowly for only 3 minutes.

3   Tip in the rice and stir gently but thoroughly, until all the grains are mixed with the vegetables. Spoon in enough of the hot stock to moisten the rice and vegetables. Continue cooking slowly until the liquid is absorbed, then add some more.

4   Season the mixture and add the peas. If the sun-dried tomatoes were in oil they can be added at this stage. Continue cooking the risotto, adding the hot stock with sun-dried tomatoes gradually. Towards the end of the cooking time, add the parsley and walnuts. Taste and adjust the seasoning.

5   When the rice is tender and just pleasantly moist, stir in the butter. The cooking time should be approximately 30 minutes.

6   Spoon onto warmed plates and top with parsley and cheese.

Variations:

- *If using frozen peas, add them towards the end of the cooking time.*
- *Add about 225g (8oz/1½ cups) well-drained canned or cooked chickpeas instead of the walnuts or use 225g (8oz/1½ cups) shelled peas.*
- *Change the selection of vegetables according to the season.*

Barley Risotto: use 170g (6oz/¾ cup) pearl barley instead of the rice in the recipe above. Blanch the barley by putting it in cold water to cover, bring the water to the boil then strain. The barley is then ready to use. Continue as the risotto above, adding the barley at stage 3. Cook for about 30 minutes or until the vegetables and barley are soft. You may find that the barley does not absorb quite as much stock as the rice.

Freezing: not recommended.

light dishes

 The recipes that follow are quick to prepare and ideal for lunch or supper. Most of the recipes are based on eggs, as these provide an ideal basis for light meals at any time of the day.

oeufs à la tripe SERVES 4

Onions are one of the important vegetables to include in your diet. You can choose mild or strongly flavoured onions for this dish. If you want an even milder taste, substitute shallots, leeks or even spring onions (scallions) for ordinary onions.

Ingredients

METRIC (IMPERIAL)		AMERICAN
5	large eggs	5
30g (1oz)	butter	2 tablespoons
1 tablespoon	olive oil	1 tablespoon
225g (8oz)	onions, finely chopped	2 cups
2 level tablespoons	cornflour (cornstarch)	2½ level tablespoons
570ml (1 pint)	milk	2½ cups
to taste	sea salt and freshly ground white pepper	to taste
to taste	grated or ground nutmeg	to taste

To garnish

chopped hard-boiled (hard-cooked) egg

chopped parsley

Method

1 Hard-boil the eggs. Plunge into cold water to cool them rapidly, then crack and remove the shells.

2 Heat the butter and oil in a saucepan. Add the onions and cook gently for 5 minutes, stirring from time to time so they do not brown.

3 Blend the cornflour (cornstarch) with the onions, then gradually add the milk, stirring or whisking as it comes to the boil and the sauce thickens. Lower the heat and allow the sauce to simmer gently for 10 minutes. Season and add the nutmeg.

4 Slice 4 of the eggs, add to the hot onion mixture and heat for 1 or 2 minutes only. Spoon into individual dishes. Chop the fifth egg and spoon over the top of each dish, sprinkling with chopped parsley.

Serve with a spoon and fork.

Variations: if you are anxious to avoid butter then use all olive oil. When cooking the onions in a non-stick saucepan, or in a bowl in the microwave, you can manage with just the 1 tablespoon olive oil and no extra fat.

Freezing: not recommended as the eggs become very rubbery.

eggy bread SERVES 1

This dish, which was a feature of the days of egg shortages, is an interesting way to get the nutritional benefit of eggs.

Ingredients

METRIC (IMPERIAL)		AMERICAN
1	slice of bread	1
1	egg	1
to taste	sea salt and freshly ground black pepper	to taste
	For frying	
30g (1oz)	butter	2 tablespoons

Method

1   Cut the slice of bread into fingers. Break the egg onto a large plate, whisking until yolk and white are mixed, then season lightly.
2   Gently heat the butter in a large frying pan (skillet) then dip the fingers of bread into the beaten egg. Make sure the fingers are coated on both sides but do not soak for too long or they will break.
3   Lower the coated fingers into the hot butter and cook for 1 minute or until the egg has set. Turn over and cook on the other side for the same time. Serve at once.

Variations:
*   *Use olive oil instead of butter to cook the bread.*
*   *If you use gluten-free bread, the egg coating makes it much more palatable.*

Freezing: not recommended.

pipérade SERVES 3–4

The additional ingredients in this recipe give scrambled eggs flavour, colour and extra nutrients. Make sure the vegetables are tender, but not over-soft, before adding the eggs so they retain their moist texture. Although the pepper can be cooked without removing the skin, the flavour is better if this is done. The term 'concassed', below, means the tomatoes are skinned, halved, deseeded and chopped finely. This step is not essential but it gives a smoother mixture.

Ingredients

METRIC (IMPERIAL)		AMERICAN
1	green (bell) pepper	1
55g (2oz)	butter or margarine	¼ cup
1	medium onion, finely chopped	1
1	garlic clove, finely chopped	1
2	tomatoes, concassed	2
6	large eggs, whisked	6
to taste	sea salt and freshly ground black pepper	to taste

Method

1 Halve the pepper and discard the core and seeds. To remove the skins, place the pepper halves under a preheated grill (broiler) with the rounded sides uppermost and leave until the skin turns black. Place in a plastic bag, leave until quite cold then strip away the skin. Chop the pepper flesh into small pieces. If you do not skin the pepper, simply discard the core and seeds and chop the flesh finely.

2 Heat the butter or margarine, add the onion and cook gently for 3 minutes. Put in the garlic, pepper and tomatoes. Cook slowly for about 6 minutes or until soft.

3 Add the eggs, mixing with the vegetables. Season to taste and gently stir until the eggs are set to personal taste. Serve on hot toast or on a bed of cooked rice or lentils. Pipérade is good served cold with a salad of watercress and uncooked fennel.

Variations:

- *Add grated or finely chopped, diced Cheddar or other good cooking cheese with the eggs, together with finely chopped basil or parsley. Goat's cheese is particularly good with the eggs.*
- *Heat chopped prawns (shrimp) in the butter or margarine, add the beaten eggs and scramble.*
- *Heat diced carrots, fennel or globe artichoke hearts before adding eggs and scrambling.*

Freezing: not recommended as the eggs become very rubbery.

omelettes

An omelette is an 'easy-to-eat' egg dish that can be varied almost endlessly. Herbs can be added to the eggs or the omelette can be filled with savoury or sweet ingredients. The water is not essential but it makes a lighter dish.

Ingredients

METRIC (IMPERIAL)		AMERICAN
2	large eggs	2
to taste	sea salt and freshly ground black pepper	to taste
1–2 tablespoons	water, optional	1–2½ tablespoons
30g (1oz)	butter or olive oil	2 tablespoons
	To garnish	
	parsley or any vegetables	

Method

1 Beat the eggs lightly, add the seasoning and the water. Heat the butter or oil in the omelette pan. About half of this can be tipped into the eggs immediately before cooking. This gives the omelette more flavour.

2 Pour the eggs into the omelette pan. Leave for a very short time until the bottom has set, then tilt the pan so the liquid egg runs from the top to the sides. Continue like this until the omelette has set, then fold it away from the handle and tip onto a warmed plate. Garnish and serve.

Variation: another way of working the omelette, which some people prefer, is to move the eggs as they set, rather as though making scrambled eggs, then finally allowing the omelette to form a good shape.

FLAVOURING PLAIN OMELETTES

Aux fines herbes: add a selection of finely chopped herbs, including those recommended on the diet, such as basil, dill, fennel leaves, mint and parsley. Mellow-tasting Roast Garlic (*see page 142*) could be added to the beaten eggs or used as a filling.

With cheese: either add finely grated Cheddar or any low-fat cheese to the eggs or fill the omelette with soft cream or curd cheese before folding. Chopped herbs blend well with cheese, so these can be included.

With chicken: fill the omelette with diced or minced chicken in horseradish-flavoured live yoghurt or a sauce, such as the Watercress Sauce (*see page 151*), before folding.

With fish: fill the omelette with flaked, cooked fish, such as salmon or white fish, in dill- or fennel-flavoured live yoghurt or Watercress Sauce (*see page 151*).

With vegetables: cooked, diced globe artichoke hearts make a delicious filling for the omelette, as do creamed carrots (mashed with a little olive oil and chopped basil).

Freezing: not recommended.

soufflé omelettes SERVES 1

While this very light type of omelette is generally served as a dessert, there is no reason why it cannot be a savoury dish and flavoured in exactly the same way as the examples given on pages 176–7.

Ingredients

Use the same ingredients as on page 176, but milk could take the place of the water. The eggs can be seasoned or lightly sweetened, depending upon the flavouring.

Method

1 Separate the eggs. Beat the yolks with seasoning or 1–2 teaspoons sugar. Add the water or milk.

2 Whisk the whites in a separate bowl until they form soft peaks, then fold into the yolks. Preheat the grill (broiler) on a medium setting.

3 Heat the butter or olive oil in the omelette pan, pour in the eggs and cook steadily until the bottom of the omelette is just set. The top will still be soft and runny. Do not work it as the plain omelette.

4 Place the omelette pan under the grill (be careful not to burn the handle) and cook steadily until the eggs are set. Spoon the filling over half the omelette, fold away from the handle and tip onto a warmed plate. Serve at once. The omelette can be topped with sifted icing (confectioner's) sugar before serving.

FILLINGS FOR SWEET SOUFFLÉ OMELETTES

These fillings can be hot or cold.

Apricots and Almonds: mix a thick purée of cooked apricots with a little honey and finely chopped almonds.

Apple and Ginger: flavour thick, sweetened apple purée with a crushed gingernut biscuit or chopped stem ginger or a good pinch of ground ginger. The apples can be flavoured with lime or lemon juice and sweetened with honey.

Banana and Walnut: mash a banana with a little live yoghurt and add chopped walnuts.

Berry Fruits: fill with mixed uncooked or cooked, lightly sweetened berry fruits, such as blueberries, raspberries and sliced strawberries.

Note: sprigs of mint can be used as a decoration, or a little chopped mint can be added to the egg yolks. Mint blends well with fruit.

Freezing: not recommended.

a slice of toast

Sometimes a slice of toast, spread with butter or a chosen alternative, is just what you want. When you fancy a change, however, here are some suggestions:

- *Make the toast interesting by choosing a different type of bread. Multigrain bread is both delicious and nutritious.*
- *Rye is one of the grains recommended for a healthy gut. Rye bread, often sold as pumpernickel, tastes completely different to wheat bread and breaks easily. Rye crispbreads are another alternative.*
- *Supermarkets sell a selection of Italian breads, which make good toast. Like most British breads, they are made from wheat.*
- *Most breads contain gluten. If you have a gluten intolerance, buy gluten-free bread. These days, most gluten-free loaves taste good and toast well.*
- *Cornbread has become very popular, although the yeast type does contain a high percentage of wheat flour.*

EASY TOPPINGS FOR TOAST

All of these can be used without spreading butter, or an alternative, on the toast.

Apple: grate raw apple and mix with grated raw carrot, moistening with a few drops of yoghurt or milk. Mix the pulp of baked, cooled apple with finely chopped dates or raisins and/or chopped almonds.

Banana: mash with a few drops of lime or lemon juice. Baked Bananas (*see page 201*) can be mashed and served hot or cold.

Cheese: mix soft cheese with chopped dates or other dried fruit, including ready-to-eat apricots or prunes or chopped nuts. Also try mixing soft cheese with chopped basil, mint or parsley. Grate hard cheese and mix with a little Mayonnaise (*see page 157*).

Chicken: mix finely minced, cooked chicken or other poultry or meat with a little home-made Mayonnaise (*see page 157*).

Dates: if fresh, they will be sufficiently soft to be stoned and finely chopped to make a spread. If dried, chop and mix with a little live yoghurt or low-fat soft cheese.

Fish: pound cooked kipper or mackerel or salmon flesh until smooth. Moisten with a few drops of virgin olive oil and flavour with lime or lemon juice and a shake of pepper or pinch of ground ginger.

Fruit: various fresh fruit purées are excellent spreads. Make a thick purée in a food processor or liquidizer (blender). Sweeten acid fruit with a little honey, but do not make the purée too sweet as it should be refreshing.

Garlic: to make a bruschetta, rub the hot toast with a cut garlic clove then moisten with a generous amount of virgin olive oil. To turn this into a complete main dish, top with salad ingredients and portions of chicken, meat, fish, lentils or chickpeas. Roast Garlic (*page 142*) is another good savoury topping. Ciabatta or other Italian breads are ideal but any bread could be used.

Ginger: spread the toast with the syrup from preserved stem ginger and top with finely chopped stem ginger.

Honey: look for the organic type. Thick honey is more suitable than thin.

Horseradish: spread a very thin layer of the sauce or horseradish cream over the toast.

Pâté: the Liver Pâté on page 95 makes an excellent spread, as do most kinds of pâté. If buying ready-made, check it is very fresh and buy organic pâté if possible.

Preserves: jams, jellies, marmalades and even some chutneys make good spreads for toast. Choose low-sugar preserves when possible. Maple syrup is another choice; add a squeeze of lemon juice to lessen its sweetness.

Sardines: mash cooked or canned fish.

Watercress: this is delicious with butter, but finely chopped watercress leaves are sufficiently soft to use as a spread when mixed with a few drops of virgin olive oil.

Butter Plus

Butter, or an alternative spread, is given more flavour if mixed with other ingredients.

Anchovy Butter: mix butter with finely chopped or flaked fish, or a few drops of anchovy essence, together with a little lime or lemon juice.

Herb Butter: choose herbs that are important for a healthy gut, blending a generous amount with butter. Basil, dill, fennel, lemon balm, mint and parsley are particularly pleasant.

Nut Butter: blend chopped nuts with butter. Peanut butter is a great favourite but, before serving, check that people are not intolerant or even allergic to this.

Seed Butter: blend a small amount of seeds, such as caraway, cardamon, cumin, dill, fennel, poppy or sesame, with butter. Most seeds have a strong flavour, so use sparingly. Sprouting seeds like alfafa are an excellent addition to the diet.

desserts

Even if you rarely make a dessert it is worth doing so for anyone who is trying to cure, or alleviate, gut trouble. A dessert is generally easier to eat than a more substantial main course. Desserts should be based on nourishing and recommended ingredients that play a real part in helping the gut (*see pages 54–5*). The recipes that follow have been chosen to produce easy-to-digest, tempting dishes.

yoghurt lemon syllabub SERVES 4

A syllabub is one of the oldest British traditional recipes. Originally, it was far more liquid than the dessert we know today. By using live yoghurt with a small amount of whipped cream, you will create a dessert with a similar texture to the syllabubs of the old days, although much lighter and less fattening.

Ingredients

METRIC (IMPERIAL)		AMERICAN
1–2	lemons*	1–2
115g (4oz) or to taste	loaf (lump) sugar	¼lb or to taste
140ml (¼ pint)	white wine	⅔ cup
425ml (¾ pint)	live yoghurt, as thick as possible	scant 2 cups
140ml (¼ pint)	double (heavy) cream, whipped	⅔ cup

* Choose unwaxed lemons.

Method

1   Wash the lemons in cold water and dry well. Rub the lumps of sugar over the surface of the fruit to extract the very top zest. If you have no lumps of sugar then finely grate the top zest and use 115g (4oz/½ cup) caster sugar. The zest gives a very strong flavour so, if you are not over-fond of a sharp, lemony taste, do not use too much. Halve the fruit and squeeze out the lemon juice.

2   Put the lemon-coated sugar, or lemon zest and caster sugar, with the wine into a basin, and allow it to stand until the sugar has dissolved.

3   Fold into the yoghurt then add the whipped cream. Taste the mixture and incorporate as much lemon as desired. Spoon into individual glasses or dishes. Chill well before serving.

Variations:

*   *If you require a more generous amount of cream then replace some of the yoghurt with whipped cream.*
*   *Use fromage frais instead of some of the yoghurt.*

Apple Syllabub: omit the lemon zest and most of the juice and use 230ml (8fl oz/1 cup) cooked apple purée. Sweeten to taste.

Banana Syllabub: use a little lemon juice but omit the lemon zest and add 2 smoothly mashed bananas.

Other Flavourings: use mashed raspberries or other soft fruit or a thick purée of cooked apricots or plums or uncooked pears or mangoes.

Freezing: not recommended.

cranachan SERVES 4–6

Cranachan is a traditional Scottish dessert. One of the main constituents is oatmeal – an excellent source of soluble fibre needed to prevent constipation (see pages 61–3). For this dish the oats are toasted, which gives them a delicious nutty taste. The traditional recipe uses a large amount of whipped cream, but live yoghurt is used here instead to cut down on fat.

Ingredients

METRIC (IMPERIAL)		AMERICAN
85g (3oz)	rolled oats	scant I cup
285ml (½ pint)	live yoghurt	1⅓ cups
I tablespoon	honey	I tablespoon
225g (8oz)	fresh raspberries	½lb
1–2 tablespoons	whisky, preferably Drambuie	1–2½ tablespoons

Decoration
extra raspberries

Method

1. There are two ways of toasting rolled oats. You can spread them in a layer in an ungreased heavy frying pan (skillet) and heat them slowly on top of the cooker, turning them over several times. The second method is to spread the rolled oats in one flat layer on a baking tray and heat them for 10–12 minutes in a preheated oven set to 180°C/350°F/Gas Mark 4 or 160–170°C with a fan oven. The rolled oats should be just golden; if too dark they tend to acquire a slightly bitter taste. Allow to cool completely before using. Toasted oats can be stored in an airtight tin or jar.
2. Mix the yoghurt with the honey. Blend in the oats, half the raspberries and the whisky.
3. Spoon the remaining raspberries into sundae glasses and top with the oat mixture. Decorate and chill well before serving.

Variations:

- *Tofu can be used in place of the yoghurt. Process in a liquidizer (blender) with the honey.*
- *Use other soft berry fruits, such as sliced strawberries, whole blueberries, blackberries or loganberries.*

Freezing: not recommended.

ice cream SERVES 6–8

Ice cream is wonderfully tempting when you are not completely fit and perhaps not feeling particularly hungry. This recipe is based on an egg custard and cream. It can be adapted to make it less rich (see 'Variations').

Ingredients

METRIC (IMPERIAL)		AMERICAN
3	large eggs	3
55g (2oz) or to taste	caster sugar	¼ cup or to taste
425ml (¾ pint)	milk	scant 2 cups
I	vanilla pod (bean) or ½ teaspoon vanilla extract*	I
425ml (¾ pint)	double (heavy) cream	scant 2 cups

* This has a better flavour than vanilla essence.

Method

1 Break the eggs into a bowl, whisk in the sugar and then add the milk with the vanilla pod or extract. Either pour into the top of a double saucepan or leave in the bowl. Stand over a pan of hot, but not boiling, water and cook until sufficiently thick to make a good coating over a wooden spoon. Stir briskly or whisk while cooking. Cover and allow the custard to get quite cold. Remove the vanilla pod – this can be rinsed in cold water, dried and used again or placed in a jar of sugar to flavour it.

2 Whisk the cream until it stands in soft peaks, fold in the strained cold custard, pour into a container and freeze.

Variations:

*   *Use half double (heavy) cream and half full-cream yoghurt.*

With an ice cream maker: there is no need to separate the egg whites as the mixer aerates the ingredients as it freezes them. You can be more economical and use single, instead of double, cream or half cream and half live yoghurt.

Fruit Ice Creams: these are excellent for encouraging people to eat more of the recommended fruits (*see page 54*). Blend equal quantities of whipped double cream and thick fruit purée together and sweeten to taste. Try a purée of melon and bananas, apples and lime, mixed soft berries or other fruits as they come into season.

Spiced Ice Cream: incorporate some of the spices suggested on page 55, such as ground cinnamon or ginger. This makes the ice cream appealing to anyone who likes stronger flavours.

Freezing: do not make the ice cream mixture too sweet or it will be too soft and difficult to freeze. The basic version of the Ice Cream or a Fruit Ice Cream can be stored in the freezer for up to 4 weeks, but the version containing full-cream yoghurt or the economical version is better eaten with a week. Remove from the freezer about 10 minutes before serving and place in the refrigerator.

melon and citrus sorbet SERVES 4–6

A fruit sorbet (sherbert) enables you to incorporate a whole range of fruits in a most refreshing form. In this recipe, the melon purée blends well with the sharp flavour of the citrus fruits.

Ingredients

METRIC (IMPERIAL)		AMERICAN
I	medium-sized melon (about 800g/1¾lb before peeling)	I
285ml (½ pint)	orange juice	1⅓ cups
2 tablespoons	lemon juice	2½ tablespoons
I tablespoon	lime juice	I tablespoon
2 tablespoons	honey or caster sugar	2½ tablespoons

Method

1 Halve the melon, scoop out and discard the seeds and remove the pulp. Put this with the other ingredients into a liquidizer (blender) or food processor and process until you get a smooth mixture.

2 Pour into an ice cream-making tray or suitable container and freeze until lightly frosted.

3 Remove the sorbet from the freezer and spoon into a bowl. Whisk briskly to aerate the mixture, then return it to the container and continue freezing.

Variations:

*   *Use watermelon instead of an ordinary melon.*
*   *Use any mixture of fruits that are in season. Berry fruits are wonderful for summer. While cooked fruits could be used, select uncooked fruit if possible.*
*   *Fruit juices make good sorbets.*

To make a lighter mixture: fold 1 or 2 whisked egg whites into the fruit, after whisking it as stage 3 (you will be using uncooked eggs). Alternatively, soften 2 level teaspoons gelatine in 2 tablespoons cold orange juice (extra to that given in the recipe), then dissolve over hot water. Add to the other ingredients, then freeze.

With an ice cream maker: these are perfect for making light, well-aerated sorbets. Simply tip the smooth purée, made as stage 1, into the ice cream maker and switch on to freeze. There is no need to use gelatine or egg whites.

Freezing: sorbets can be stored for up to 6 weeks. Bring out of the freezer about 15 minutes before serving.

empress rice SERVES 4–6

This dish is made with a rice pudding and an egg custard. These two are combined, and gelatine added, to produce an unusual cold dessert. The extra ingredients – dates, apricots and nuts – not only add to the food value but also make it suitable for a special occasion. Use ready-to-eat dried apricots. Organic ones have a better flavour but are not as brightly coloured as fruit that has been treated.

Ingredients

METRIC (IMPERIAL)		AMERICAN
85g (3oz)	short-grain (pudding) rice	scant ½ cup
850ml (1½ pints)	milk	3¾ cups
55g (2oz)	caster sugar	¼ cup
¼ teaspoon	almond extract	¼ teaspoon
2	large eggs	2
15g (½oz) sachet	gelatine	1 envelope
2 tablespoons	sweet sherry	2½ tablespoons
3 tablespoons	sieved apricot jam	3¾ tablespoons
3 tablespoons	finely chopped dates	3¾ tablespoons
3 tablespoons	finely chopped apricots	3¾ tablespoons
3 tablespoons	blanched chopped almonds	3¾ tablespoons
140ml (¼ pint)	double (heavy) cream, whipped	⅔ cup

Method

1. Put the rice with 570ml (1 pint/2½ cups) of the milk, half the sugar and the almond extract into the top of a double saucepan or in a basin. Cook over a pan of boiling water for 30–35 minutes or until the grains are tender.

2. Meanwhile, whisk the eggs with the remaining sugar, add the rest of the milk and stir over hot, but not boiling, water until the mixture is sufficiently thickened to coat the back of a wooden spoon.

3. Add gelatine to the cold sherry. Allow to stand for 3 minutes then add to the hot rice pudding and stir over a gentle heat until the gelatine has dissolved.

4. Strain the hot egg custard into the hot rice pudding and add the apricot jam. Allow the mixture to cool completely, cover and place in the refrigerator until it stiffens slightly (this is important as it means the dates, apricots, nuts and cream will remain suspended in the soft pudding).

5   Fold in the dates, apricots and almonds and lastly half the whipped cream. Spoon into a 1.2 litre (2 pint/5 cup) mould or a number of individual moulds and leave to set. Turn out and top with the remaining cream.

Freezing: not recommended.

rice pudding SERVES 4

Rice is an ideal food for people suffering from intestinal complaints because it contains no gluten and provides easily digestible complex carbohydrates. You may not have had old-fashioned rice pudding for some time but I am sure you will enjoy it by itself or served with your favourite fruit. Make certain you buy the right kind of rice – short-grain (pudding) type – as this will make a lovely, creamy pudding.

Ingredients

METRIC (IMPERIAL)		AMERICAN
55g (2oz)	short-grain rice	good ⅓ cup
570ml (1 pint)	milk	2½ cups
2 tablespoons	honey or sugar*	2½ tablespoons
30g (1oz)	butter, optional	2 tablespoons
1 teaspoon	ground cinnamon	1 teaspoon

*You can alter the taste of the pudding by your choice of sugar, so vary this from time to time, using caster, granulated, Demerara or light Barbados sugar.

Method

1 Preheat the oven to 140–150°C/275–300°F/Gas Mark 1–2 or 120–130°C with a fan oven.

2 Place the rice, milk and sugar into a 1.2 litre (2 pint/5 cup) pie dish. Cut the butter into small pieces, if using, and mix with the other ingredients.

3 Top with the ground cinnamon and bake for 2½–3 hours. Serve hot.

Freezing: not recommended.

Note: stirring the pudding after about 1 hour adds to the creamy texture. In this case, add the cinnamon topping after stirring.

Variation:
Rice Custard: whisk 1 or 2 large eggs, add the milk and then strain this liquid over the rice in the dish.

rice soufflé pudding

This turns a rice pudding into a special dish, full of nourishing ingredients.

Ingredients

METRIC (IMPERIAL)		AMERICAN
55g (2oz)	short-grain rice	good ⅓ cup
570ml (1 pint)	milk	2½ cups
3 tablespoons	caster sugar	scant 4 tablespoons
about 5	lemon balm leaves or strips of lemon zest	about 5
30g (1oz)	butter	2 tablespoons
2	large eggs	2

Method

1 Put the rice, milk, 1 tablespoon of the sugar, the lemon balm or lemon zest and the butter into the top of a double saucepan or a large basin and cover.

2 Place over a saucepan of simmering water and cook for 35–40 minutes or until the rice is tender and the pudding has become thick and creamy.

3 Remove the lemon balm leaves or lemon zest.

4 Preheat the oven to 170°C/325°F/Gas Mark 3 or 140–150°C with a fan oven.

5 Separate the eggs. Whisk the yolks into the hot rice mixture. Whip the whites until they stand up in peaks, whisk in the remaining sugar then fold the whites into the rest of the ingredients.

6 Spoon into a buttered 18cm (7 inch) soufflé dish and bake for 25–30 minutes or until well risen and firm. Serve hot with a purée of fruit.

Freezing: not recommended.

banana and pear crumble SERVES 4–5

A fruit crumble is an exceptionally easy hot pudding to make and a delicious combination of flavours and textures. Bananas, pears and dates are fruits that provide good amounts of fibre and nutrients needed for a healthy gut (see Chapter 4). Use fresh dates if they are available, otherwise the dried variety will do.

All fruits in this recipe are firm, so orange and lemon juices are added to provide extra moisture.

Ingredients

METRIC (IMPERIAL)		AMERICAN
	Fruit layer	
2	large bananas, peeled and sliced	2
2	ripe but firm medium pears, peeled, cored and sliced	2
4 tablespoons	chopped dates	5 tablespoons
2 tablespoons	orange juice	2½ tablespoons
I tablespoon	lemon juice	I tablespoon
	Crumble topping	
85g (3oz)	butter or margarine	⅜ cup
170g (6oz)	plain (all-purpose) flour	1½ cups
½–I teaspoon	ground cinnamon	½–I teaspoon
85g (3oz)	caster sugar	⅜ cup

Method

1. Preheat the oven to 180°C/350°F/Gas Mark 4 or 150–160°C with a fan oven.
2. Put the fruit with the orange and lemon juices into a 1.2 litre (2 pint/5 cup) pie or oven-proof dish. Make sure the fruit is levelled on top to give a good base for the crumble mixture. Cover the dish with foil and cook for 5 minutes only, then remove the foil.
3. Rub the butter or margarine into the flour, adding the cinnamon and sugar. Sprinkle on top of the fruit, giving an even layer. Return to the oven and bake for 30 minutes or until the topping is golden in colour. Serve with live yoghurt.

Freezing: not recommended as these particular fruits tend to become over-soft.

pineapple and apple crisp

This is an adaptation of the Flapjack recipe on page 214. The crisp oatmeal topping makes an excellent change from a fruit crumble. Do not over-sweeten the fruit base as you need a contrast to the sweetness of the oatmeal mixture.

Ingredients

METRIC (IMPERIAL)		AMERICAN
	Topping	
55g (2oz)	butter or margarine	¼ cup
55g (2oz)	soft brown sugar	¼ cup
2 level tablespoons	golden (corn) syrup	2½ level tablespoons
140g (5oz)	rolled oats	1½ cups
30g (1oz)	plain (all-purpose) flour	¼ cup
	Fruit layer	
455g (1lb)	cooking apples, weight when peeled, cored and sliced	1lb
225g (8oz)	fresh pineapple, weight when skinned and finely diced	½lb
2 tablespoons	water	2½ tablespoons
1–2 tablespoons	soft brown sugar	1–2½ tablespoons

Method

1 Put the butter or margarine, sugar and syrup into a saucepan and melt over a low heat. Remove from the heat and stir in the rolled oats and flour. Mix thoroughly and cool slightly as the mixture becomes easier to spread over the fruit when cool.

2 Preheat the oven to 180°C/350°F/Gas Mark 4 or 140–150°C with a fan oven.

3 Put the apples, pineapple, water and sugar into a 1.2 litre (2 pint/5 cup) pie dish. Cover with a little foil and cook for 10 minutes. Remove the foil and make sure the fruit is spooned into a flat base.

4 Spoon the oatmeal mixture over the top of the fruit, spreading with the back of a metal spoon to form a smooth layer.

5 Bake for 30 minutes or until golden brown. Serve hot with live yoghurt.

Freezing: not recommended.

welsh eve's pudding SERVES 4–6

English Eve's pudding consists of a sponge baked over apples. I have chosen the Welsh version, Pwdin Efa, because it is more interesting. Apples are one of nature's most healing foods, and you can read more about them in Chapter 4.

Ingredients

METRIC (IMPERIAL)		AMERICAN
680g (1½lb)	cooking apples	1½lb
140ml (¼ pint)	water	⅔ cup
55g (2oz)	caster sugar	¼ cup
	Topping	
55g (2oz)	butter or margarine	¼ cup
55g (2oz)	plain (all-purpose) flour	½ cup
340ml (12fl oz)	milk	1½ cups
few drops	vanilla extract	few drops
30g (1oz)	caster sugar	2 tablespoons
3	large eggs	3

Method

1 Peel and slice the apples, put into a saucepan with the water and sugar and cook gently until a fairly smooth purée.

2 Spoon into a greased 1.2 litre (2 pint/5 cup) pie, soufflé or other ovenproof dish. Meanwhile, preheat the oven to 180°C/350°F/Gas Mark 4 or 160–170°C with a fan oven.

3 Heat the butter or margarine in a good-sized saucepan, stir in the flour and cook, stirring well, over a slow heat for 2–3 minutes. Add the milk and vanilla extract, stirring or whisking as the sauce comes to the boil and thickens. Add the sugar and remove from the heat. Cool slightly.

4 Separate the eggs. Beat the yolks into the warm sauce. Whisk the egg whites until very stiff and fold into the ingredients in the saucepan. Spoon the light mixture over the apples.

5 Bake for 40 minutes or until well risen and golden. Serve at once.

Variation: spoon the apples and then the topping into individual deep, ovenproof dishes, such as soufflé dishes. Bake for approximately 20 minutes or until well risen and golden.

Freezing: not recommended.

baked apples SERVES 4

Baked apples may seem a very simple dessert but they are a splendid way of enjoying the concentrated flavour of the fruit. The thick, smooth pulp from baked apples makes an ideal filling for the Soufflé Omelette on page 178 as well as other dishes.

Although some dessert apples, such as Cox's, can be baked, the right kind is a good cooking apple, such as a Bramley, which makes a fluffy pulp. Choose good-sized fruit.

Ingredients

METRIC (IMPERIAL)		AMERICAN
4	cooking apples, each about 225g (8oz/½lb)	4
	filling, optional (*see below*)	

Method

1 Wash the apples in cold water and dry thoroughly. Preheat the oven to 180°C/350°F/Gas Mark 4 or 140–150°C with a fan oven.
2 Remove the core of the apples with a special apple corer or a small, sharp knife. Slit the skin around the centre. These steps prevent the pulp bursting through the skin.
3 Stand the fruit on an ovenproof dish, add the filling (*see below*) if required and bake for approximately 50 minutes. Serve hot with live yoghurt or custard.

FILLINGS FOR BAKED APPLES

- *Chopped dates, by themselves or with a little lemon, lime or orange juice to soften them.*
- *Chopped dried apricots, moistened with lemon, lime or orange juice. Use the ready-to-eat type and choose organic fruit if possible.*
- *Honey and chopped almonds, pine nuts or walnuts.*

In addition you could have:

- *butter and brown sugar*
- *raisins or other dried fruit*
- *mincemeat*

- *apricots or other jams or jellies: bramble jelly is particularly good*
- *golden (corn) or maple syrup*

Variations:

Microwave 'Baked' Apples: prepare the fruit in exactly the same way as for oven baking. The apples cook in a very short time: 1 large apple takes about 4 minutes on full output. Cooking several apples at once takes longer. The exact timing will vary with the fruit and the output of the microwave so check in your microwave instruction book.

The flavour of the fruit is excellent but the skins tend to be tougher than when the apples are baked in the oven. If you have a combination microwave, however, the skins will be perfectly soft.

Barbecued 'Baked' Apples: prepare the fruit as above, adding a filling if desired. Wrap each apple separately in foil to make a package. Stand on a metal baking tin over the barbecue fire and cook for about 50 minutes. Always open the foil carefully as steam builds up inside.

Freezing: do not freeze the whole cooked fruit, although apple purée freezes well.

baked bananas

Bananas are an excellent source of easily digested carbohydrates, fats and potassium needed for normal fluid balance and muscle activity. Eaten raw or cooked, they contribute to a healthy diet. The fruit is delicious baked in its skin and served hot. Cooked bananas have an entirely different taste and texture to raw ones.

Preheat the oven to 190°C/375°F/Gas Mark 5 or 170–180°C with a fan oven. Put the unpeeled fruit into an ovenproof dish and bake for 18–20 minutes, depending on the size of the bananas. The skin will turn very dark. Do not over-bake or the juice tends to seep through the skin and the pulp loses its moist texture.

Bananas can also be cooked in the microwave. In this case prick the skin two or three times and put the fruit into a microwave dish. One banana takes 1½–2 minutes on full output. The skin may split slightly, even when pricked. Several bananas will take longer.

Always take care when peeling cooked bananas as both the skins and fruit are very hot.

Freezing: not recommended.

sweet accompaniments

fruit

As you will see from reading Chapter 4, various fruits have special healing benefits that help maintain gut health. Undoubtedly the simplest, and one of the best, ways to enjoy fruit is to eat it raw. This may not appeal to everyone, and certain fruits do need cooking.

Serve a fruit salad as often as possible, selecting fruits from the list of healthy gut foods on page 54. Apples and pears are always a good choice.

fruit coulis SERVES 4

The term 'coulis' refers to a clear, unthickened sauce. A coulis can be either savoury or sweet, but one based on fruit is an ideal accompaniment to a rice pudding or ice cream. This recipe with kiwi fruit has a refreshing taste and is an excellent source of vitamin C.

Ingredients

METRIC (IMPERIAL)		AMERICAN
6 tablespoons	water	7½ tablespoons
I tablespoon	caster sugar or clear honey	I tablespoon
6	ripe kiwi fruit	6

Method

1 Put the water and sugar or honey into a small saucepan and heat until the sugar has dissolved. This can also be done in a bowl in the microwave. Allow to cool.

2 Halve the kiwi fruits and remove all the pulp. Add to the syrup, then sieve or liquidize to give a smooth sauce.

Variations:

*   *Raspberries and other ripe, soft fruit can be used in the same way. Use less water if the fruit is very juicy.*

*   *Fruit that needs some cooking, such as firm apricots and blackcurrants, should be simmered in the water and sugar but never over-cooked.*

Freezing: a coulis freezes well.

baking

The recipes that follow will enable you to prepare some interesting and easy-to-make dishes that the whole family will enjoy. They include ingredients included in the list of healthy gut foods on pages 54–5. Sometimes someone who is unwell does not eat much food for lunch, so they will be ready for a home-made scone, biscuit or slice of cake at teatime.

To ensure perfect results it is important to weigh and measure ingredients carefully and to ensure the oven is properly preheated before baking. If you have any doubts about the accuracy of your oven temperature it is worth investing in an oven thermometer. If you have just acquired a fan oven, be prepared for the cooking time to be a little shorter than when baking in a standard oven, so do check baking progress early.

Do not change the basic proportions in the recipes as these have been carefully tested to give a good result. You can increase or decrease the amount of spices, however, as they are a matter of personal taste.

USING DIFFERENT KINDS OF FLOUR

If you are anxious to include some of the grains recommended on page 55, you can use small amounts in the basic scone recipe (*overleaf*). Instead of 225g (8oz/2 cups) of wheat flour, use just 170g (6oz/1½ cups) of wheat flour plus 55g (2oz/½ cup) barley flour or rye flour. Do not exceed these amounts.

- *If using plain flour, use exactly the same amount of baking powder.*
- *If using self-raising flour, sift this with ¼ teaspoon baking powder.*
- *The barley or rye flour should be sifted with the wheat flour.*
- *Cornmeal or polenta are not suitable for scones.*
- *Rice flour is excellent in biscuits but gives too dry a texture in scones.*
- *Many good supermarkets sell these different flours, as do health-food shops.*

scones MAKES FROM 8 (see stage 3)

Home-made scones (biscuits), whether sweet or savoury, are an ideal way to tempt the somewhat fickle appetite of anyone who is not completely fit. A freshly baked, light scone may be more appealing both to the eye and the appetite than slices of bread or toast.

The recipe begins with basic sweet scones, ideal for teatime or throughout the day. This is followed by suggested variations, including recipes for savoury scones, which are an excellent accompaniment to soups, cheese or light main dishes.

The important points to remember when making scones, are:

a. Make the dough appreciably softer than for pastry.
b. Do not over-handle the dough before shaping. You can pat out the dough, rather than using a rolling pin.
c. Bake at a high temperature and test early so the scones are not over-baked and become dry as they cool.

If the person with gut trouble has been recommended a special spread, rather than butter or margarine, make sure it is suitable for baking.

Ingredients

METRIC (IMPERIAL)		AMERICAN
225g (8oz)	self-raising flour or plain (all-purpose) flour with 2 teaspoons baking powder	2 cups
pinch	sea salt	pinch
30–55g (1–2oz)	butter or margarine or recommended spread	2 tablespoons to ¼ cup
55g (2oz) or to taste	caster sugar	¼ cup or to taste
140ml (¼ pint)	milk, see stage 2	⅔ cup

To glaze
milk or 1 beaten egg

Method

1 Preheat the oven to 220°C/425°F/Gas Mark 7 or 200–210°C with a fan oven. With this basic recipe there is no need to grease the baking tray; a light dusting of flour makes sure the scones do not stick. With most variations you should either grease the tray or line it with baking parchment.

2 Sift the flour, or flour and baking powder, with the salt. Rub in the butter or margarine or spread; do not over-handle the dough. Add the sugar then gradually incorporate the milk. While full-cream milk makes richer scones, skimmed milk could be used. Makes of flour vary, so add the last drops gradually. The dough should be soft but not too sticky.

3 Turn on to a lightly floured surface and roll or pat until about 2cm (¾ inch) thick. Cut into the required size with a pastry cutter. When people are unwell it may be wise to make really small rounds. Place on the baking tray. To give an attractive shine, brush the tops with milk or egg.

4 Bake for 10–12 minutes. To test if cooked, press at the sides of the scones; they should feel just firm to the touch. Lift on to a wire cooling tray. If you want them crisp on the outside, do not cover. If you prefer a soft scone, place a teacloth (kitchen towel) over them.

Freezing: it is important to freeze the scones when just cold as they then retain their freshly baked taste when defrosted. You could warm them by putting them in a hot oven for 1–2 minutes.

Variations: mix the scone dough with half milk and half live yoghurt. This produces a very light scone.

Gluten-free flour: this makes good scones. Follow the quantities as in the basic recipe and the suggestions that follow.

Olive Oil Scones: add 1 tablespoon olive oil to the sifted flour. You will need less milk to bind the mixture together. Do not exceed this amount of oil.

SWEET SCONES

Almond: add 55g (2oz/⅓ cup) blanched, chopped almonds to the flour. When the scones are shaped, brush with milk or beaten egg and top with more chopped almonds. You could also add dried fruit as in the following suggestions.

Apricot: add 1 teaspoon finely grated lemon zest to the flour as well as 55g (2oz/⅓ cup) finely chopped, ready-to-eat, dried apricots. Buy organic ones if you can.

Citrus Fruits: add 1 or 2 teaspoons finely grated lemon or orange zest to the flour. Mix the dough with a little lemon or orange juice in place of some of the milk.

Dates: this dried fruit is important on the diet. Add about 115g (4oz/⅔ cup) finely chopped dates with the sugar. Other dried fruits, such as raisins, can be used.

Ginger: sift 1 teaspoon ground ginger with the flour then add 2 or 3 (2½ to scant 4 tablespoons) finely chopped, preserved or crystallized ginger with the sugar (*see also under 'Savoury Scones'*).

Oatmeal: use 55g (2oz/½ cup) less flour and add the same amount of rolled oats instead. Use the same amount of baking powder with plain flour and add ½ teaspoon baking powder with self-raising flour. Dried fruit such as almonds, apricots and dates can be added to oatmeal scones. Savoury Oatmeal Scones can also be made. Omit the sugar and add a generous amount of seasoning to the oatmeal. Chopped herbs are an excellent addition.

SAVOURY SCONES

Omit the sugar in the basic recipe and sift the salt plus a good shake of freshly ground black pepper with the flour. You could also add ½–1 level teaspoon mustard powder.

Basil: this is a very important herb on the diet and gives a pleasing flavour. Add 2 tablespoons finely chopped basil to the flour. Other herbs, as recommended on pages 54–5, can be used instead.

Cheese: add 55g (2oz/½ cup) finely grated Cheddar or other good cooking cheese to the mixture, after rubbing in the fat. A tablespoon chopped herbs, such as parsley, basil or coriander (cilantro), can also be added.

Cumin: add 2–3 teaspoons cumin seeds after rubbing in the fat. Blanched almonds or raisins blend well with the seeds; add 2–3 tablespoons (2½ to scant 4 tablespoons). Cumin scones are a particularly good accompaniment to soups.

Garlic: add 1–2 finely chopped garlic cloves, after rubbing in the fat. For a milder taste, use Roast Garlic (*see page 142*). The garlic is then fairly soft, so adjust the amount of liquid accordingly. Instead of garlic, you could use 3–4 tablespoons (scant 4–5 tablespoons) very finely chopped chives or spring onions (scallions).

Ginger: use 2.5–3.5cm (1–1½ inches) peeled then grated or very finely chopped root ginger. Add to the mixture after rubbing in the fat. A small amount of basil or other chopped herbs could be used as well.

apple muffins

Apples contribute healing substances to food when used in both sweet and savoury dishes. American-style muffins have become very popular, and can be served at any time of the day. Do not over-beat this muffin mixture; just combine the ingredients quite gently.

The recipe assumes you are using stiff pulp from baked apples (see page 199). If stewing the fruit, use a small amount of water only and no sugar and follow the adaptation under 'Variations'.

Ingredients

METRIC (IMPERIAL)		AMERICAN
115g (4oz)	butter	½ cup
200g (7oz)	apple purée	1 cup
55g (2oz)	sultanas (seedless white raisins) or dried figs, very finely chopped, optional	⅓ cup
200g (7oz)	plain (all-purpose) flour	1¾ cups
2 level teaspoons	baking powder	2 level teaspoons
pinch	sea salt	pinch
1 teaspoon	allspice or ground ginger	1 teaspoon
1	large egg	1
1½ tablespoons	milk	2 tablespoons

Method

1 Preheat the oven to 200°C/400°F/Gas Mark 6 or 180–190°C with a fan oven. Grease small muffin tins (pans) or bun tins well or insert paper cases into the tins.

2 Put the butter with the apple purée into a saucepan or basin and heat until the butter has melted; this could also be done in the microwave. Add the sultanas or figs to the warm mixture; this helps to soften the dried fruit.

3 Sift the flour, baking powder, salt and allspice or ginger together. Beat the egg with the milk.

4 Blend the dry ingredients with the apple mixture then add the egg and milk, stirring gently. Do not worry if the mixture looks slightly lumpy.

5 Spoon into the prepared tin or paper cases and bake for 15–20 minutes, depending on size. The muffins should be just firm. Over-baking makes them too dry. Serve while warm or freshly baked.

Variations:

- *If using smooth stewed apple purée, omit the milk in the recipe.*
- *Apricots or figs could be used; stew the fruit until a smooth, thick purée. Use the same weight as for apples. Follow the recipe above but omit the milk.*
- *Use 200g (7oz/1 cup) mashed ripe bananas with 2 (2½) tablespoons lemon or orange juice or milk.*

Berry Muffins: use 140g (5oz/1 cup) whole raspberries or blueberries with 1½ (2) tablespoons milk.

Freezing: these freeze well. Warm gently after defrosting to restore their fresh flavour.

Gluten-free flour: if you are baking for someone who has been advised to avoid ordinary wheat and other grains because of gluten content, use gluten-free plain flour and follow the recipe above. You should get very good results.

gingernut biscuits MAKES 16-18

Ginger is packed with healing substances useful in controlling nausea and other health complaints. The rather unusual baking instructions for these biscuits ensure that the mixture spreads out correctly and forms the small cracks that are a feature of these famous biscuits.

Gingernuts are sometimes used to thicken a stew, instead of flour. Simply break 2 or 3 into small pieces, add to the cooked, hot stew and leave for a short time for them to break into smaller pieces, then stir briskly to blend into the liquid.

Ingredients

METRIC (IMPERIAL)		AMERICAN
55g (2oz)	butter or margarine	¼ cup
2 tablespoons	golden (corn) syrup	2½ tablespoons
30g (1oz)	caster or soft brown sugar	2 tablespoons
115g (4oz)	plain (all-purpose) flour	1 cup
½ teaspoon	bicarbonate of soda (baking soda)	½ teaspoon
½–1 teaspoon or to taste	mixed spice	½–1 teaspoon or to taste
1 teaspoon	ground ginger	1 teaspoon

Method

1 Preheat the oven to 200°C/400°F/Gas Mark 6 or 180–190°C with a fan oven. Grease 2 or 3 baking trays.

2 Put the butter or margarine, syrup and sugar into a large saucepan, stir over a low heat until the ingredients have melted, then remove from the heat.

3 Sift the flour with the bicarbonate of soda and the spices, add to the melted ingredients and mix thoroughly. Allow to cool enough to handle.

4 Gather up pieces of the mixture and roll into 16–18 small balls. Place on the baking tray, allowing plenty of space between the balls for the mixture to spread.

5 Bake for 5 minutes only at the setting given in stage 1, then reduce the heat to 170°C/325°F/Gas Mark 3 or 140–150°C with a fan oven and bake for a further 10 minutes or until golden brown. If your electric oven holds the heat for a long time, switch it off and let the biscuits cook in the residual heat.

6 Cool on the baking tray for 10 minutes, then lift onto a wire cooling rack. When quite cold, store in an airtight tin away from other biscuits.

Variation: use maple syrup instead of golden syrup.

Freezing: this is not necessary as the biscuits keep well in a tin.

apricot triangles MAKES 8–10

This recipe produces small cakes with a crisp, biscuit-like texture. Use tender, ready-to-eat dried apricots. These, with the rolled oats, are an excellent way to boost the amount of constipation-fighting soluble fibre in your diet.

Ingredients

METRIC (IMPERIAL)		AMERICAN
85g (3oz)	butter or margarine	⅜ cup
85g (3oz)	dried apricots, finely chopped	⅜ cup
55g (2oz)	sultanas (seedless white raisins)	⅓ cup
85g (3oz)	rolled oats	scant 1 cup
85g (3oz)	sugar, preferably Demerara	⅜ cup
55g (2oz)	self-raising flour or plain (all-purpose) flour with ½ teaspoon baking powder	½ cup
1	large egg, whisked	1

Method

1 Put the butter or margarine into a large bowl and stand this over a pan of boiling water to melt. This can also be done in the microwave.

2 Add the apricots and sultanas to the hot fat; this tenderizes the dried fruit. Leave until quite cold before adding other ingredients.

3 Preheat the oven to 180°C/350°F/Gas Mark 4 or 160–170°C with a fan oven. Line the base of a 23–25cm (9–10 inch) round sandwich tin (layer pan) with baking parchment or greased greaseproof paper. Grease the sides of the tin.

4 Add the rolled oats, sugar, sifted flour, or flour and baking powder, then the egg to the ingredients in the bowl. Mix thoroughly.

5 Spoon into the prepared tin and smooth flat on top. Bake for 30–35 minutes or until golden and firm to the touch.

6 Cool the cake for a few minutes, then mark into triangles while warm. Leave in the tin until almost cold, then carefully remove. These cakes keep fresh for 2–3 days in an airtight tin. Store away from other cakes or biscuits.

Freezing: open freeze then pack.

flapjacks MAKES ABOUT 12

Oatmeal is a healthy food because it helps prevent constipation, but did you know it also helps control levels of blood cholesterol? Make use of it wherever possible. Flapjacks are a favourite with young and old, so these are likely to be very popular. Both ground cinnamon and ginger are highly recommended so you can choose which spice to incorporate into the other ingredients. Butter gives the best results in these biscuits.

Ingredients

METRIC (IMPERIAL)		AMERICAN
85g (3oz)	butter	⅜ cup
55g (2oz)	caster sugar	¼ cup
2 tablespoons	golden (corn) syrup	2½ tablespoons
I teaspoon	ground cinnamon or ground ginger	I teaspoon
170g (6oz)	rolled oats	scant 2 cups

Method

1 Preheat the oven to 190°C/375°F/Gas Mark 5 or 170–180°C with a fan oven. Grease an 18cm (7 inch) square sandwich tin (layer pan). Do not line it with greaseproof paper or baking parchment.

2 Put the butter, sugar and syrup into a saucepan and heat until the ingredients have melted. Remove from the heat and stir in the spice and rolled oats.

3 Tip the mixture into the tin and spread flat. Bake for 25 minutes or until evenly golden brown. Leave for about 3 minutes, then mark the mixture into fingers. Do not try and remove these from the tin at this stage or they will break.

4 When almost cold, lift the biscuits onto a wire cooling tray. When quite cold, store in an airtight tin away from other biscuits.

Freezing: not recommended.

Variations: a 20cm (8 inch) tin could be used to give thinner biscuits. Reduce the baking time by about 5 minutes.

Almond Flapjacks: as almonds are an excellent food for gut disorders, add 2 (2½) tablespoons finely chopped almonds at the end of stage 2.

date rascals MAKES ABOUT 24 CAKES

The following recipe is based on a traditional British cake. Instead of the usual currants and raisins, however, I have included dates because of their mild laxative effect and high energy content. These small, crisp cakes are an ideal way to tempt the appetite.

Ingredients

METRIC (IMPERIAL)		AMERICAN
225g (8oz)	self-raising flour or plain (all-purpose) flour with 2 teaspoons baking powder	2 cups
pinch	sea salt	pinch
115g (4oz)	lard (shortening) or butter	½ cup
85g (3oz)	caster sugar	⅜ cup
85g (3oz)	dried dates, finely chopped	½ cup
1	large egg, whisked	1
few drops	water or milk	few drops

Method

1 Preheat the oven to 200°C/400°F/Gas Mark 6 or 180–190°C with a fan oven. Lightly grease two baking sheets (tins) or line with baking parchment.

2 Sift the flour, or flour and baking powder, with the salt into a mixing bowl. Rub in the lard or butter until the mixture is like fine breadcrumbs. If using a food processor or electric mixer, do not over-mix.

3 Add the sugar, dates and then the egg, mixing well. Gradually stir in just enough water or milk to make a rolling consistency.

4 Roll out the dough until about 1.5cm (½ inch) thick then cut into 5cm (2-inch) rounds. Place on the baking trays and cook for 13–15 minutes or until golden. Lift onto a wire cooling tray. Eat when freshly baked.

Variation: substitute 55g (2oz/good ½ cup) rolled oats for the same amount of flour. In this case sift just ½ level teaspoon baking powder with the self-raising flour. Use the same amount of baking powder with plain flour.

Freezing: these freeze very well; open freeze, so they do not stick together, then pack.

ginger carrot cake

Both carrots and ginger are included in the list of healthy gut foods on page 54. Carrots provide fibre, minerals and vitamins, and ginger helps calm a nervous digestive system. Combined in this delicious recipe, they provide an inviting means of ensuring a healthy gut. Ground ginger is used as the flavouring in this cake, and luxurious preserved ginger in the topping.

Peel or scrape the carrots just before making the cake so they are kept moist. Never place whole or grated carrots in water as that would incorporate too much liquid into the cake mixture.

Ingredients

METRIC (IMPERIAL)		AMERICAN
	For the cake	
170g (6oz)	butter or margarine	¾ cup
170g (6oz)	caster or light brown soft sugar	¾ cup
3	large eggs, whisked	3
170g (6oz)	self-raising flour or plain (all-purpose) flour with 1½ teaspoons baking powder	1½ cups
1–2 teaspoons or as required	ground ginger	1–2 teaspoons or as required
170g (6oz)	carrots (weight when grated)	1⅔ cups
55g (2oz)	blanched almonds, chopped	½ cup
	For the topping	
55g (2oz)	soft cream cheese	¼ cup
30g (1oz)	butter or margarine	2 tablespoons
55g (2oz)	icing (confectioner's) sugar, sifted	½ cup
3 tablespoons	sliced preserved ginger	scant 4 tablespoons

Method

1 Preheat the oven to 190°C/375°F/Gas Mark 5 or 170–180°C with a fan oven. Grease and flour the cake tin (pan) or line it with greased greaseproof paper or baking parchment.

2 Cream the butter or margarine and sugar until soft and light, then gradually beat in the eggs. Sift the flour, or flour and baking powder, with the ground ginger; fold into the creamed ingredients with the carrots and nuts.

3 Spoon into the tin and bake for 1 hour or until firm to the touch. Allow to cool in the tin for 10 minutes, then turn out onto a wire cooling tray. Leave until quite cold.

4 Cream the cheese, butter or margarine and icing sugar together. Spoon over the top of the cake. Cover with the preserved ginger.

Freezing: open freeze, then pack.

Variations:

*   *Instead of butter or margarine use 170ml (6fl oz/⅔ cup) olive oil and stir into the other ingredients. This makes a good cake but the texture is not as light as when creaming the fat with the sugar.*
*   *Use only 115g (4oz/1 cup) self-raising flour and 55g (2oz/½ cup) ground almonds. In this case, sift ½ teaspoon baking powder with the flour. If using plain flour, add 1½ teaspoons baking powder as in the recipe above.*

smoothies

The word 'smoothie' describes a mixture of fruits, with some herbs and even a few vegetables, yoghurt or milk formed into a smooth drink. A smoothie is thicker than a juice but should never be so solid that it is difficult to drink. When someone is not completely fit, often it is an effort to eat solid food, and this is when a smoothie is a sensible alternative.

I am not giving set recipes with quantities, as smoothies are purely a matter of personal taste and a wise use of the ingredients available. Instead, I have suggested some very pleasing combinations of flavours. When making smoothies, boost their flavour and healing benefits by including some of the healthy gut foods (pages 54–5) as ingredients.

Smoothies have become so popular that special machines are available, but an ordinary liquidizer (blender) is excellent for the purpose. A food processor can also be used, but do not fill this too generously or some of the soft mixture could seep down around the cutting blade.

TO MAKE SMOOTHIES:

1   Add the ingredients to the goblet or food processor bowl. Do not over-fill. Put on the lid, switch on at a medium speed, process until all the ingredients begin to soften, then increase the speed. Hold the lid firmly in position when using a liquidizer because the mixture rises in the goblet.

2   If the blades do not revolve easily, it means the mixture is a little too stiff. Add a small amount of liquid then switch on again.

3   With a smoothie machine, you turn the tap and let the mixture flow into a jug or individual glasses. With a liquidizer, remove the lid and tip the goblet so the mixture can be poured into a jug or glasses. With a food processor, it is wise to place the bowl on a large plate before removing the lid and central blade. If any liquid does run down the central hole, it can be spooned up from the plate.

4   Serve the smoothie cold. A very little crushed ice could be put into the glasses, but check this is allowed on the diet. Too much ice would spoil the flavour. Smoothies can also be served warm, but do not over-heat.

SUGGESTED SMOOTHIE COMBINATIONS

You do not have to select a large number of ingredients. A smoothie can be made with just one ingredient but the following examples produce most interesting flavours. Aim for an attractive colour as well as a delicious flavour.

Remove bitter pith from citrus fruit, peel and core from apples and pears, and any large pips or stones.

Autumn Special: diced pears and dessert apples with lemon or lime juice and live yoghurt. This can be given a spicier flavour by adding a little stem ginger or ginger wine.

Citrus Special: orange and pink or ordinary grapefruit segments, orange or tangerine juice, banana(s) plus a little honey if required to sweeten.

Cool Green: diced melon, kiwi fruit, white grapes, lime juice.

Exotic Special: fresh figs, melon, lime, pinch ground ginger.

Golden Smoothie: orange segments, grated young carrots, skinned and deseeded tomatoes, a few basil leaves.

Richly Dark: blueberries, blackberries, a few chopped dates, red wine.

Summer Berries: raspberries, redcurrants, strawberries, banana(s), live yoghurt, shredded mint leaves.

Vegetable Special: a few spinach leaves, grated young carrots, tender celery heart, pine nuts, a little single cream or live yoghurt.

refreshing drinks

Well-chosen drinks are important when you want to maintain a healthy gut (see Chapter 4). Water and the liquid from fresh fruit are ideal too. With modern gadgets you can extract juice from a great variety of fruits and from juicy vegetables. In addition to these, here are some very refreshing drinks.

Appleade: wash about 455g (1lb) apples but do not peel or core them. Cut into small pieces and put into a large container with several strips of lemon zest. Pour 570ml (1 pint/2½ cups) boiling water over the apples and lemon zest and press the fruit with a wooden spoon. Leave until cold, then strain the liquid and add the juice of 1 lemon and any sweetening required. This juice can be diluted with water.

Variation: ripe pears could be used instead of apples.

Lemonade: grate the top zest from 2 well-washed lemons and put into a jug. Pour 570ml (1 pint/2½ cups) boiling water over the zest. Leave until cold, then strain and add the juice from 2 lemons and any sweetening required. Warm for a few minutes to dissolve the sugar. This juice can be diluted with water.

Variations: use 2 limes or 3 oranges in place of the lemons, or try a mixture of citrus fruits.

Fresh Milk Shake: put a few spoonfuls of soft fruit, such as raspberries, chopped strawberries or a mixture, into a liquidizer. Add a tumbler of cold milk and switch on until blended. You can choose semi-skimmed milk or any of the other milks you prefer (see page 92). The drink can be made richer by adding a small spoonful of ice cream with the fruit.

Variation: vary the milkshakes with any seasonal fruit available.

Ginger Milk Shake: follow the directions for Fruit Milk Shake but add diced stem or preserved ginger instead of fresh fruit.

Mint Tea: this is famous in Arab countries, where it is served hot and sweetened. It is delicious with less sugar and can be served hot or cold. Put about 10 small mint leaves into a small teapot or larger beaker. Add about 285ml (½ pint/1⅛ cups) boiling water. Press the leaves with a spoon then strain and serve hot or well chilled.

Variations:

- *Use other herbs, such as camomile, lemon balm, basil, tansy or rosemary.*
- *A little lemon or lime juice can be added to the strained liquid.*

Milk Tea: if you have been advised to increase your intake of milk, try making tea with boiling skimmed milk or a mixture of milk and water instead of the usual boiling water.

Iced Tea: strain your favourite tea, allow it to become very cold, then serve over crushed ice. Add a little lemon juice and/or a few sprigs of mint for extra flavour.

Iced Coffee: if coffee is included in your diet, try the beverage iced. Make the coffee in the usual way, cool and pour over crushed ice. Top with a little whipped cream.

Variation: make ultra-strong coffee, cool and pour into an ice-making tray. Place in the freezer. Put 1 or 2 cubes of the iced coffee into a tumbler and fill with ice-cold milk. Top with whipped cream.

Pineapple Wine Cup: this is a drink for a special occasion that everyone can share. Peel a small fresh pineapple, cut into dice and discard the hard centre. Put into a chilled bowl. Top with 2 bottles dry white wine and flavour with a little lemon juice. Decorate with rings of cucumber and sprigs of mint.

appendix one
good food hygiene

 Food poisoning caused by bacterial or viral contamination is the most common cause of vomiting and diarrhoea.

Nasty bacteria lurking in a bowl of creamy potato salad or hiding in a sandwich filling can result in painful and frequent trips to the toilet. The time from consuming tainted food to the first symptoms of nausea or diarrhoea can be amazingly swift – often only a matter of a few hours. Contaminated food is eaten, dangerous bacteria or viruses infect the gut and multiply at an amazing rate, and toxins are released; these signal to the brain and internal organs that a washing-out is needed. After that the victim has little control. Once this natural, but unpleasant, cleansing process is completed, the victim usually suffers little more than feeling 'delicate' while the body restores its fluid balance, and a new bloom of normal gut bacteria is established (*see page 23 for information about probiotics*).

This scenario can, however, have a different ending. *E-coli* and *salmonella* are examples of bacteria well known for causing outbreaks of diarrhoeal illness. *Botulism* is a less well-known but potentially fatal bacterial invader. An anaerobic organism that grows in poorly sterilized bottles and cans of food, botulism produces a toxin so dangerous it can be used as a biological weapon. Other examples of dangerous bacteria include *listeria* (danger foods are soft cheese and meat pâté) and *cryptosporidium* (a parasite that can contaminate both foods and water). Pregnant women, the elderly and people with damaged immune systems should take strict precautions to avoid these organisms.

To understand the health and economic implications of food poisoning, all we need do is recall the problems caused by the bacteria group salmonella. Since the 1980s the rise in contamination of poultry products – especially eggs – has resulted in increasing numbers of cases of food poisoning and extensive costs to farmers.

Major advances have been made within the food industry to control the problem of contamination. Strict laws have been enacted governing hygiene in places of food production, points of sale and eating establishments. But that alone cannot resolve the problem. While it is true that a dodgy curry served in a scruffy local can be the source of infection, we are more prone to illness from foods prepared at home. In fact, cases of food poisoning from meals eaten at home are on the increase, especially during the warm summer months.

What can be done? Paying more attention to basic food hygiene at home is the answer.

the danger foods

Eggs: Remember that salmonella continues to infect egg-laying flocks. Unless you choose eggs that carry the Lion mark (showing that they are from flocks of birds known not to carry salmonella), eat hard-boiled eggs and avoid mayonnaise and other foods made with uncooked eggs.

Poultry: Contamination of poultry with salmonella and campylobacter bacteria is the consequence of intensive farming, and can cause diarrhoea (lasting for several days), headaches, nausea and vomiting. To avoid these problems, thaw frozen poultry completely, cook until no pink can be seen around the bone and the internal temperature is at least 80°C (176°F). The juices of well-cooked poultry run clear. As for stuffing a bird, try lightly filling the internal cavity with fresh herbs and slices of apple, and bake the stuffing in a separate dish.

Follow the rules of good kitchen hygiene as you prepare poultry, wash your hands frequently, and avoid touching foods that will not be cooked – green salads and ice cubes, for example.

Soft-rind cheeses: Unpasteurized foods may carry Listeria monocytogenes, which can cause serious medical consequences, including damage to unborn children. Know the source of what you buy, and avoid these foods if you are pregnant or have a damaged immune system.

Pork: Cook until the meat has lost all its pink colour. Raw or undercooked pork may be infested with trichinosis (a parasite) that can cause serious illness, so cook until the internal temperature is at least 75°C (176°F).

Rules for safe food at home

1. Always remove your rings because bacteria lurk under them and in their detailed faceted work.
2. Wash down work surfaces before and after food preparation.
3. Wash your hands with soap and hot water thoroughly and often during meal preparation. Raw poultry and meat are prime suspects for infection, so be sure to wash your hands well after handling these products.
4. Use separate chopping boards for cooked and raw foods. These should be well washed in running water after each use – a quick wipe-down is not enough!
5. Knives used to cut poultry, meat or fish should be washed after each use with soap and hot water.
6. Keep your refrigerator and freezer at the temperatures recommended by the manufacturer. Buy a thermometer for each appliance and check its temperature from time to time. Keep the interior of your appliances clean.
7. Keep food in the refrigerator. Opened cans and bottles, leftovers (especially rice), custards and mayonnaise, meat, fish and poultry are excellent breeding grounds for bacteria.
8. Keep all foods well covered and store in an appropriate place in the refrigerator. Bag or wrap raw poultry, meat and fish, and store where they cannot drip fluid onto foods that are not going to be cooked before eating, such as salads and custards.
9. Fresh fruit and vegetables – especially those used in salads – should be well rinsed under cold running water.

Beef: Unless you know the source of your beef and eggs – and know that the meat was recently ground – avoid steak tartar, as it is an excellent harbour for both E. coli and salmonella.

10. Prepared bags of salad greens are a popular choice these days, but watch out for bacteria! Rinse greens well in running water before eating.

11. Inspect canned foods before you use them. Discard any tin or bottle with a bulging top, because this is a sure sign the contents are infected with dangerous bacteria (*see the comments about botulism, above*). Discard rusty or dented cans, and always rinse the top of a tin before opening it.

12. Never reheat foods more than once in an oven or microwave.

13. Thaw frozen foods completely before cooking unless the product label gives instructions for cooking from frozen. It is best to thaw meat, fish and poultry in the refrigerator – less damage is done to the product, and there is less chance of bacteria multiplying where the food is no longer frozen.

14. Immediately clean up food and drink spilt on the kitchen floor.

15. Ban pets from the kitchen. Cats, dogs and all other lovable creatures carry bacteria than can cause serious infections.

16. If your gut is susceptible to infection (for example, if you have recently taken a course of antibiotics, or if you have a damaged immune system), particular attention should be given to soft fruit, such as strawberries and grapes, and raw vegetables. Some experts believe you can help remove bacteria and any chemical residues by rinsing these foods in plenty of running water and then letting them rest for about 10 minutes in a large bowl of fresh water to which 1 or 2 tablespoons of vinegar have been added.

appendix two
medication and your gut

If gastrointestinal problems suddenly develop, consider whether or not you have recently begun a course of medication. A change in contraception, for example, may trigger bowel problems. And many of us know from experience that antibiotics taken to cure a bacterial infection can upset the delicate balance of normal bacteria in the gut, resulting in soft stools and diarrhoea. Other common reactions to medication include constipation and nausea. Some drugs, such as aspirin and ibuprofen, can even cause gastric bleeding if taken over an extended period.

What to do about physical problems caused by essential medication presents a real quandary. The advice in Chapter 4 about foods that help control specific gastric and bowel conditions can help you live comfortably with your medication. If symptoms do not respond, you will need to seek other help. Start with your local pharmacy, but if symptoms include signs of blood, a fever or severe gastric pain, tell your doctor at once.

medications that commonly cause gut symptoms

NON-STEROIDAL MEDICATION

These drugs are often used to treat pain and inflammation caused by injury, arthritis and gout, and include aspirin, ibuprofen, fenbufen, mefenamic acid and piroxicam.

The vast majority of people experience no side-effects from these medications, but they can cause nausea, indigestion, diarrhoea and – in extreme cases – erosion of the stomach lining that may develop into an ulcer. If you are taking these products and experience digestive problems, discuss them with your doctor.

ANTIBIOTICS

In the few decades since the discovery of the miracle of antibiotics, uncounted millions of people have been saved from deadly bacterial infections. Like all powerful drugs, however, antibiotics may cause side-effects, the most common of which are nausea, diarrhoea or a rash.

Antibiotics work by targeting and killing specific groups of bacteria; unfortunately, sometimes the normal bacteria in a healthy gut are also affected. (As discussed in Chapter 2, a balance of healthy bacteria is required for the gut to work.) When this balance is disturbed, the result can be a surge in the presence of unwanted flora in the gut and the sudden onset of symptoms. If this occurs, a good first response is to try to re-establish the presence of normal gut flora by increasing your intake of live yoghurt and probiotics products (*see page 23*).

Dangerous allergic reactions to antibiotics can occur, with symptoms of itching, facial swelling and breathing difficulties. If any of these conditions develop, seek medical help at once.

ANTI-CANCER DRUGS

Early reactions to anti-cancer drugs include nausea, vomiting and diarrhoea. For advice about which foods can help control these symptoms, see the relevant sections in Chapter 5.

ANTACIDS

Antacids can cause gastric symptoms. For example, products containing magnesium may cause diarrhoea, while those containing aluminium may cause constipation. Some people taking sodium bicarbonate for gastric problems may experience flatulence.

The efficiency of some medications can be impaired by antacids. For this reason, always tell your doctor if you are taking them.

LAXATIVES

Excessive use of laxatives can cause diarrhoea and dependency, so only take these products when truly needed. They can also cause flatulence and abdominal pain. The best way to maintain a normal active bowel is to include high-fibre foods – such as wholegrain cereals and root vegetables – in your daily diet.

Never include laxatives as part of a weight-loss programme.

LIPID-LOWERING DRUGS

Some drugs in this category affect the way in which the gut responds to fats in the diet. They can limit the absorption of fat-soluble vitamins (*see page 236*), and vitamin supplements may be needed. Ask your local pharmacist or doctor for guidance.

seeking help from a pharmacist

As a practical approach, your local pharmacist is a good place to start seeking help when you are unwell. Choosing from a wide range of over-the-counter products can be very confusing, and if you are in doubt about which product best suits your needs, ask for help. Many people fall into the trap of selecting a product based on advertisements they have seen. Just because the manufacturer claims a product works does not mean it is the right one for you. Qualified pharmacists are highly trained members of the health-care community, and they can discuss your specific symptoms and guide you through the maze of packages and containers. They will also ask important questions about other medications you may be taking, and explain how you should best use a new product.

When talking to the pharmacist, remember to be factual about your problem. Many people are put off talking to a pharmacist because the conversation takes place in public and may be overheard, unlike the privacy of a doctor's office. Little help can be given if the facts of your condition are not known – so be discreet but honest when you describe your problem. Always tell the pharmacist about other medications you are taking, as this will help them select the best product for you. If possible, get all your medications from the same pharmacy. Over time they will come to know your needs and specific medical problems.

Remember: if the pharmacist suggests you should see your GP, follow that advice.

prescription drugs from your doctor

Medication prescribed by your doctor will work only if taken as directed. Failure of a drug to cure a problem frequently results from three factors: a patient fails to complete the course of medication due to improvement in symptoms; there is a misunderstanding about instructions given with the drug; or the patient has a fear of adverse reactions.

Always read the patient information leaflet included in the packaging. If an information sheet is not included with your prescription, ask your pharmacist for one. Read the entire sheet, giving special attention to side-effects. Most pharmaceuticals have side-effects on occasion – most are mild, but in some cases serious conditions can result. Reading the information sheet will tell you which symptoms are common and mild, and which should be reported to your doctor. Do not panic when you read the list of side-effects! They usually include all possible conditions, including the rarest. Rest assured that the chances are you will take your medication with no ill effects.

Report all medication you take when questioned by your doctor – that includes both over-the-counter and prescribed drugs. He or she may also wish to know which dietary supplements you take, as these can have important physiological effects; for example, depending on the amount taken, fish oil may thin the blood. This would be important information if you were on blood-thinning drugs, such as warfarin.

When you get a new prescription from your doctor, make certain you know the name of the drug, why you are taking the drug, how much to take, the frequency and times of day it should be taken, if it should be taken on an empty stomach or with a meal, whether or not alcohol will lower its effectiveness, and how long you should continue the course of medication. Write this information down and put it in a handy place. This may sound a little too simple, but you would be surprised how many people are so anxious during an appointment with their doctor that they totally forget what they have been told.

It is a good idea, while you are with the doctor, to ask about possible side-effects. If you have a tendency to suffer from diarrhoea, for example, and this may result from taking your new medication, ask your doctor for a means of countering this symptom.

Safety rules for taking medication

- Keep medications in a safe place away from children.
- Use only according to directions on the label; read these carefully.
- Always return unused medications to a pharmacy for destruction.
- Never take medicine from unlabelled containers.
- Never give your medication to someone else.
- Make certain your prescription is labelled clearly. Many people find adding a small label of their own to the packaging helps them remember what each drug is for, but never allow this to cover the label applied by the pharmacist.
- Take tablets and capsules with water when you are in a standing or upright position.
- Measure your dose carefully – keep a 5ml spoon and a measured medicine cup on hand. If you are using a dropper, count the drops carefully.
- Shake the bottle before measuring out a dose of a liquid drug.
- You may need to avoid certain foods when taking a medication – acidic fruit juice, for example, may reduce the effect of certain antibiotics; dairy products may hinder absorption of certain medications.
- Terrible-tasting medicine can be washed down with a drink of water. You cannot over-dilute a swallowed dose.
- Instructions about when you should take medication can be confusing: four times a day usually means that it should be taken four times during waking hours, but ask your doctor to be sure.
- Remember: always read the label and follow the dosage on the packaging, and never take more than is recommended.

glossary

Allergens: Substances that cause allergies.

Allergies: An abnormal immune response to a harmless substance causing one or more of the following symptoms: itching (especially around the mouth), hay fever (sneezing), rash and swelling. Extreme reactions may lead to bronchospasm, anaphylactic shock and death.

Antibody: A protein produced by white blood cells in response to a specific substance, or antigen.

Antigen: A substance that stimulates the production of antibodies by the immune system.

Ayurveda: The foundation of this system of healing predates the *Veda*, the spiritual and philosophical writings of the fifth century BC, said to have been given to one or more Hindu 'seers' by the god Indra. Human life extends from the life of the creator, or 'cosmic conscience', and health is determined by the state of balance between the individual and this greater power.

In Ayurveda the body is composed of five great elements – Ether, Air, Fire, Water and Earth. At the risk of oversimplification, therapy is based on identifying and correcting imbalances among these elements. The harmony of this balance is controlled by three forces – Vata, Kapha and Pitta. Each individual has all three forces, but one dominates the others unless a state of perfect health exists. The selection of foods, how they are prepared and how they are consumed are all essentials in the search for equilibrium.

Cancer: A rampant and purposeless abnormal growth that destroys healthy tissue. Great progress has been achieved in the prevention and treatment of cancer. International experts agree that a diet rich in fruit and vegetables significantly reduces the risk of cancer within the digestive system (*see page 22*).

Cell: The smallest complete unit of life. Each cell has an external membrane, nucleus, cell fluid and small structures called organelles. To function at their best, cells must have a nutrient-rich environment provided by a healthy digestive system.

Chinese Medicine (Traditional Chinese Medicine): More than 3,000 years old, the practice of traditional Chinese medicine is still used to treat tens of millions of people. Its central theme is that humanity is part of the universe, and is therefore a small part of a greater and constant 'wholeness'. All parts of this wider creation (nature) comply with the same laws; and for humans to follow these laws is to be blessed with good health, long life and good luck. All the natural forces that shaped the universe are part of humanity, and thus part of our destiny and health.

The foundation of this healing system is the existence of two opposing forces, Yin and Yang, which together form the Tao. These forces affect all aspects of life, including the internal organ systems of the human body. Foods and herbs are categorized by the Yin and Yang system. As illness constitutes an imbalance in Yin and Yang, specific foods and herbs are prescribed in conjunction with other treatments to provide healing and restore balance.

Chronic degenerative diseases: Illnesses associated with the slow deterioration of body structures. These are often associated with the effects of ageing and include arthritis and coronary heart disease.

Digestion: The mechanical and chemical processes by which the body breaks down food into its component parts. The organs involved in this process are collectively known as the digestive system.

Elimination diet: The process of identifying specific foods, or food groups, which cause digestive sensitivity or allergic reactions in an individual.

Enzyme: A protein substance made by cells to perform a specific chemical task. Thousands of different enzymes are produced in the body.

False bleeding: The appearance of red-stained bowel motions or red staining from the rectum caused by eating fruits and vegetables containing red pigment. Beetroot is a common cause of false bleeding.

Gluten: A form of protein found in wheat, rye and barley that may cause food sensitivity and is the underlying factor in coeliac disease. Although gluten has no nutrient value for humans, it is frequently added to processed foods such as bread, canned soups, gravy granules and stock cubes to enhance the texture and appearance. People with coeliac disease should seek out products with labels clearly stating that they are gluten-free.

Helicobacter pylori: This bacterium has been identified as a factor in the development and persistence of stomach ulcers. It can be eradicated with a course of antibiotic, bismuth and specific acid-inhibitor drugs.

Inflammation/Inflammatory response: Localized pain, heat, redness and swelling that develop as part of an immune response. Increased blood flow, the concentration of fluid in an area, and the accumulation of white blood cells are involved. Inflammation is normally observed following an infection or injury.

Metabolism: The highly specific chains of chemical reactions that take place within the cells of living organisms. Metabolism involves the utilization of nutrients absorbed during digestion to produce cellular components and provide energy.

Modern medicine: The system of healing based on clinical knowledge obtained through experimentation, advanced technology and empirically derived pharmacology. Standard treatment by your GP, or in hospital, complies with the diagnostic standards and healing expectations of modern medicine.

As scientists explore and identify the value of alternative medicinal systems, modern medicine is incorporating some of their approaches into standard practice. It is no longer remarkable that a local GP might employ both homoeopathic and modern medical skills when caring for a patient.

NSAIDs: Non-steroidal anti-inflammatory drugs used to suppress pain and inflammation. Aspirin and ibuprofen are examples.

Remember: NSAIDs may encourage the formation of ulcers.

Nutrition: The balance of basic components in food that are needed for normal growth and good health. Well-balanced nutrition protects the body, whereas poor nutrition encourages disease. Poor nutrition can cause illness through dietary deficiency, or it can increase the possibility of illness by damaging the immune system and reducing the disease-resistance of body tissues.

Ulceration: The disintegration of skin or a mucous membrane to form an open sore. Most ulcers heal slowly. Causes include unusual rubbing and pressure, lack of an adequate blood supply, gastric acid (oesophagus, stomach and duodenum) and bacterial toxins.

Vitamins: A group of essential nutrients that cannot be manufactured by the human body but are present in food. The body's demand for individual vitamins varies with age, physical condition and lifestyle. Smoking, for example, greatly increases the need for vitamin C. Menstrual bleeding and childbirth increase the body's need for iron.

There are two types of vitamins: those that are soluble in water (vitamin C and all the B-vitamins are examples), and those that are soluble in oil (vitamins A, E and D).

helpful addresses and websites

British Allergy Foundation (Allergy UK)

Deepdene House, 30 Bellegrove Road, Welling, Kent DA16 3PY

Helpline: 020 8303 8583

Website: www.allergfoundation.com

British Association of Nutritional Therapists (BANT)

27 Old Gloucester Street, London WC1N 3XX

Website: www.BANT.org.uk

(Send £2 plus a self-addressed A4 envelope for a list of registered nutritional therapists.)

BBC Education: The Health Site

Online: www.bbc.co.uk//education/health

British Nutrition Foundation

High Holborn House, 52–54 High Holborn, London WC1V 6RQ

Tel: 020 7404 6504

Website: www.nutrition.org.uk

E-mail: postbox@nutrition.org.uk

Cancer BACUP

3 Bath Place, Rivington Street, London EC2A 3JR

Helpline: 0808 800 1234

Website: www.cancerbacup.org.uk

E-mail: info@cancerbacup.org.uk

Celiac Sprue Association, CSA/USA Inc.
PO Box 31700, Omaha, NE 68131–0700 (USA)
Website www.csaceliacs.org
E-mail: celiacs@csaceliacs.org

Coeliac Society
PO Box 220, High Wycombe, Bucks HP11 2HY
Helpline: 0870 444 8804
Website: www.coeliac.co.uk
E-mail: helpline@coeliac.co.uk

IBS Network
Northern General Hospital, Sheffield S5 7AU
Helpline: 01543 492192
Website: www.ibsnetwork.org.uk

Institute for Optimum Nutrition
Blades Court, Deodar Road, London SW15 2NU
Tel: 0208 877 9993

National Association for Colitis and Crohn's Disease (NACC)
4 Beaumont House, Sutton Road, St Albans, Herts AL1 5HH
Helpline: 01727 844296
Website: www.nacc.org.uk
E-mail: nacc@nacc.org.uk

NHS Direct
Tel: 0845 4647
Online: www.nhsdirect.nhs.uk

further reading

Berkson, Lindsey. *Healthy Digestion the Natural Way: Preventing and Healing Heartburn, Constipation, Gas, Diarrhoea and Gallbladder Diseases, Ulcers, Irritable Bowel Syndrome and More*, John Wiley & Sons Inc., 2000

Brewer, Dr Sarah and Berriedale-Johnson, Michelle. *Eat to Beat IBS*, Thorsons, 2002

The British Medical Association Complete Family Health Guide, Dorling Kindersley, 2000

The British Medical Association New Guide to Medicines and Drugs, Dorling Kindersley, 2001

Ewin, Jeannette. *The Plants We Need to Eat*, Thorsons, 1997

Gillie, Oliver. *Food for Life*, Hodder & Stoughton, 1998

Holford, Patrick. *Improve Your Digestion (An Optimum Nutrition Handbook)*, Piatkus Books, 2000

Lay, Joan. *Diets to Help Colitis and Irritable Bowel Syndrome*, HarperCollins, 1998

McWhirter, Alasdair and Clasen, Liz (editors). *Foods that Harm, Foods that Heal*, Readers Digest, 2002

Pitchford, Paul. *Healing with Whole Foods*, North Atlantic Books, 1993

Savill, Antoinette. *The Gluten, Wheat and Dairy Free Cookbook*, Thorsons, 2000

Sen, Jane. *Healing Foods*, Thorsons, 2001

Smith, Tony. *British Medical Association Family Doctor Series: Indigestion and Ulcers*, Dorling Kindersley, 2000

Trickett, Shirley. *Irritable Bowel Syndrome and Diverticulosis*, Thorsons, 1999

van Straten, Michael and Griggs, Barbara, *Super Foods*, Dorling Kindersley, 1990

van Vorous, Heather. *Eating for IBS*, Marlowe & Company, 2003

White, Erica. *Beat Candida Cookbook*, Thorsons, 1999

Youngson, Robert. *The Royal Society of Medicine Health Encyclopaedia*, Bloomsbury, 2000

Zinser, Stephanie. *The Good Gut Guide*, HarperCollins, 2003

38002 01127 8563

index

gluten intolerance 31, 32
  see also coeliac disease
grains 52-3, 55, 89-91
grapefruit 42
grapes 38, 46
greens 54
  adding interest 138
'grumbling appendix' 2
'gut', use of term 1, 8
gut structure 9-13

halitosis (bad breath) 74-5
Hay diet see food combining
heartburn (gastro-oesophageal reflux) 75-6
Heinz tomato soup 3
Helicobacter pylori 11, 46, 70, 72, 233
herbs 54-5, 88
hiatus hernia 76-7
high-protein diets 21
honey 46
Honey and Ginger Chicken 131
horseradish 46
Hot Watercress Sauce 151-3
Hummus 97
hygiene 85, 222-5

Ice Cream 187-8
ileum 11, 12
indigestion see heartburn
inflammation/inflammatory response 233
inflammatory bowel disease (IBD) 77
ingredients 87-92, 93
intestinal infections 34
invalid cookery 3-4, 85-6
irritable bowel syndrome (IBS, spastic colon) 5-7, 77-9

jejunum 11, 12
Jonkers, Daisy 24-5

kale 46
kiwi fruit 47

lactose (milk) intolerance 31, 32
  see also milk alternatives
Lamb Pilaf 167-8
Lamb with Barley and Caper Sauce 126-7
Lamb with Pears and Pine Nuts 128
large intestine 12
laxatives 21, 228
leeks see allium
lemons 42
Lentil Soup 110-11
lentils 47
lifestyle 28, 57
light dishes 171-82
Lime and Mint Lentil Loaf 143-4
Lime Mint Sauce 154
limes 42
lipid-lowering drugs 228
listeria 222, 224
liver (body organ) 14-15
liver (in diet) 47
Liver Pâté 95-6
Liver with Prunes and Herbs 129-30
lymphatic system 12

maize 90
malabsorption 13
malnutrition 13, 29
Mango Soup 108-9
Mayonnaise 157-8
measurements 92-3

Vinaigrette Dressing 160-1
vitamins 234
vomiting 83-4

Waldorf Salad 99
water 17-19
  requirements 19-20
watercress 52
Welsh Eve's Pudding 197-8
wheat 52-3, 91
World Cancer Research Fund 22, 23

yams 53
yoghurt 24, 53-5
Yoghurt Dressing 162-3
Yoghurt Lemon Syllabub 184-5

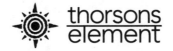